P9-EEL-976

Springer Series on the Teaching of Nursing

Diane O. McGivern, RN, PhD, FAAN, Series Editor
New York University

Advisory Board: Ellen Baer, PhD, RN, FAAN; Carla Mariano, EdD, RN, AHN-C, FAAIM, Janet A. Rodgers, PhD, RN, FAAN; Alice Adam Young, PhD, RN

Jeanne M. Novotny, PhD, RN, FAAN, is currently Dean and Professor at the Fairfield University School of Nursing. She received her Bachelor and Master of Science degrees in nursing from The Ohio State University and her PhD from Kent State University. Her career encompasses more than three decades of leadership in nursing education and administration. Dr. Novotny came to Fairfield University from the University of Virginia in 2001. She has done international work in Mexico, Chile, and Zimbabwe. Dr. Novotny holds a certificate from the Institute for Management and Leadership in Education from Harvard University and is an evaluator for the Commission on Collegiate Nursing Education. Dr. Novotny has clinical expertise in pediatric nursing and nursing leadership and has numerous scholarly publications, presentations, and consultations to her credit.

Robert H. Davis, MSN, RN, is the Director of Admissions at the Frances Payne Bolton School of Nursing at Case Western Reserve University. He has over ten years of experience in education, beginning with his role as training officer with the Lexington County Sheriff's Department teaching self-defense, pursuit driving, crime prevention, DUI detection, and D.A.R.E. Before his current role at Case, Mr. Davis was the Director of Education for Care Services, Inc., in Cleveland, Ohio, coordinating educational programs for over 1500 nursing and allied health professionals within the organization. Mr. Davis earned both his BSN and MSN in Nursing Informatics from Case Western Reserve University. He is a member of the Ohio Nurses Association and serves as their consultant to the Ohio Nursing Students' Association. He is also a member of Sigma Theta Tau, Intl.

Distance Education in Nursing

Second Edition

Jeanne M. Novotny, PhD, RN, FAAN
Robert H. Davis, MSN, RN
EDITORS

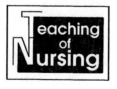

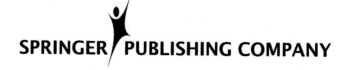

SPRINGER PUBLISHING COMPANY

Springer Publishing Company, Inc.
11 West 42nd Street
New York, NY 10036

Acquisitions Editor: Ruth Chasek
Production Editor: Jeanne Libby
Cover design by Joanne Honigman
Typeset by International Graphic Services, Inc., Newtown, PA

05 06 07 08 09 / 5 4 3 2 1

Library of Congress Cataloging-in-Publication Data

Distance education in nursing / Jeanne M. Novotny and Robert H. Davis, editors. — 2nd ed.
    p. ; cm. — (Teaching of nursing series)
  Includes bibliographical references and index.
  ISBN 0-8261-4694-5
  1. Nursing—Study and teaching. 2. Distance education.
  [DNLM: 1. Education, Nursing. 2. Education, Distance. 3. Organizational Case Studies. WY 18 D6138 2006] I. Novotny, Jeanne. II. Davis, Robert H. (Robert Henry), 1961- III. Series: Springer series on the teaching of nursing.
RT73.D56 2006
610.73'071'1—dc22   2005020835

Printed in the United States of America by Intergrated Book Technology.

Contents

Part 2: Experiences of Specific Programs

Part 3: Where Are We Going with Distance Education?

Contributors

Judith W. Alexander, PhD, MBA, RN, CNAA
Associate Professor
University of South Carolina
College of Nursing
Columbia, SC

Carolyn J. Bess, DSN, RN
Director of the RN Pre-Specialty Program
Associate Professor of Nursing
Vanderbilt University School of Nursing
Nashville, TN

Diane M. Billings, EdD, RN, FAAN
Professor, Department of Environments for Learning
Associate Dean for Teaching, Learning, and Information Resources
Indiana University
School of Nursing
Indianapolis, IN

Tracy Bushee, BSN, RN
Graduate Student
University of South Carolina
College of Nursing
Columbia, SC

John M. Clochesy, PhD, RN, FAAN, FCCM
Independence Foundation Professor of Nursing Education
Case Western Reserve University
Frances Payne Bolton School of Nursing
Cleveland, OH

Leeann Field, MA
Instructional Designer/Senior Instructor
University of Colorado at Denver and Health Sciences Center
School of Nursing
Denver, CO

Suzanne Hetzel Campbell, PhD, APRN, IBCLC
Assistant Professor
Fairfield University
School of Nursing
Fairfield, CT

Nancy Holloway, RN, PhD
University of Colorado at Denver and Health Sciences Center
School of Nursing
Denver, CO

Marcella T. Hovancsek, MSN, RN
Instructor of Nursing
Case Western Reserve University
Frances Payne Bolton School of Nursing
Cleveland, OH

Christine A. Hudak, RN, MEd, PhD
Assistant Professor of Nursing and Nurse Web Director
Case Western Reserve University
Frances Payne Bolton School of Nursing
Cleveland, OH

Pamela R. Jeffries, DNS, RN
Associate Professor of Nursing
Adult Health Department
Indiana University
School of Nursing
Indianapolis, IN

**Arlene E. Johnson, MA, RN,
  CNP**
Assistant Professor
Department of Nursing
The College of St. Scholastica
Duluth, MN

Haeok Lee, RN, DNSc
Associate Professor
University of Colorado at Denver
  and Health Sciences Center
School of Nursing
Denver, CO

Mary L. McHugh, PhD, RN, BC
Associate Professor
Director, Professional
  Development and Extended
  Studies
University of Colorado at Denver
  and Health Sciences Center
School of Nursing
Denver, CO

Kristen S. Montgomery, PhD, RN
Assistant Professor
University of South Carolina
College of Nursing
Columbia, SC

Carla L. Mueller, PhD, RN
Professor of Special Projects
School of Health Sciences
University of Saint Francis
Fort Wayne, IN

Susan M. O'Brien, EdD, RN
Dean, School of Nursing
Thomas Edison State College
Trenton, NJ

**Marilyn H. Oermann, PhD, RN,
  FAAN**
Professor, College of Nursing
Wayne State University
Detroit, MI

**Mary Ann Parsons, PhD, RN,
  FAAN**
Dean and Professor
University of South Carolina
College of Nursing
Columbia, SC

Vera Polyakova-Norwood, MEd
Distance Education and
  Instructional Support
University of South Carolina
College of Nursing
Columbia, SC

Linda Royer, RN, MPH, MSN
Assistant Professor
George Mason University
New Market, VA

Susan Stone, DNSc, CNM
President and Dean
Frontier School of Midwifery and
  Family Nursing
Hyden, KY

Tami H. Wyatt, PhD, RN
Assistant Professor
University of Tennessee
College of Nursing
Knoxville, TN

Preface

This second edition of *Distance Education in Nursing* is intended for every nurse educator from novice to expert. It addresses issues that cut across a wide spectrum of concerns related to distance education. The focus is on the impact of technology on the way that we practice nursing and, in particular, the effect of technology on how students learn. The chapters in this book give a cross section of ideas from various nursing programs across the country, as well as basic information for those who are thinking about applying some part of technology to their educational, clinical, and research endeavors.

This book has three sections. Chapters in Part 1 focus on faculty, students, and teaching strategies. Part 2 describes the experiences of specific programs, and Part 3 discusses the future of distance education.

The chapters in this second edition demonstrate the progress made in understanding the use of technology in nursing education and even more importantly the questions that need to be asked about the use of technology in the educational process. We continue to see the application of technology in our work and everyday lives and know that we could not live without it, but how we use it to improve the education of our students and the accessibility of knowledge and new competencies acquired at a distance are still questions that need answers. It is evident from the information in this book that our sophistication in the application of technology has grown immensely in the last five years.

Nurses are assuming demanding professional responsibilities related to technology in their work. These responsibilities raise important questions about the application of technology in education, clinical practice, and research for all health care professionals. Electronic information has become a central component of the practice of nursing and represents a set of challenges that, although exciting and futuristic, often seem overwhelming and frustrating. Where are we headed and what do we want from the application of technology in our educational programs, practice sites, and research endeavors?

Every nurse has a part to play in the use of technology and must be familiar with the essentials of educational formats that depend on advanced information technology. The common goal for educators, practitioners, and researchers is to expand the frontiers of knowledge in the application of technology to advance nursing science. Technology is not the focus. Rather, the use of technology to access information and knowledge that was previously inaccessible is the focus.

The content of the chapters will be useful to those interested in distance education and those who want to find ways to incorporate technology in the classroom. Research related to educational strategies and the use of technology will foster continued growth for how we educate students. We hope that you will enjoy this book and be successful in the use of technology in your teaching.

Jeanne M. Novotny
Robert H. Davis

Introduction

Susan M. O'Brien

A few days ago I was late to a statewide nursing conference. Embarrassed at being late I moved quietly, trying not to disturb others. I was surprised to be given a very warm smile by a woman already seated. Comforted by that smile I sat down, forgot my embarrassment, and became engrossed in the morning agenda. At break, my smiling neighbor leaned close to me and said, "I'm your student." Immediately my eyes dropped to her name tag. Her name opened the way for us to communicate about her work and her recent graduation from our online RN to BSN program. The conversation was warm and familiar as we discussed her plans for graduate school and her chosen area of study. Although we had never met face-to-face, we assumed an interest in each other. Another woman seated between us joined our conversation by stating she could never attend an online class because she would miss the classroom interaction. My student laughed and said that online education had more interaction than she could handle sometimes. The third woman then stated that online still would not be for her because she needed the structure of a classroom. My student confidently and expertly explained the structure of the online syllabus, the use of discussion groups, and the detail of the required assignments. The third member of the conversation listened carefully and then sighed softly. "I guess I am just old-fashioned because to me school has classrooms and people that I can see." My student then became serious and said to her neighbor and to me, "Without this online program I could never have earned a BSN. Online education made it possible to for me to go to school and juggle my many other responsibilities."

I share this story because to me it captures both the lingering attitudes toward distance education and its future possibilities. Although clearly not for everyone, distance education can open the door to lifelong learning for those who need or prefer it. Distance education has been defined as "the acquisition of knowledge and skills through mediated information and instruction, encompassing all technologies and other forms of learning at a distance" (United States Distance Learning Association, 1998). For approximately 100 years, innovative nurse educators have sought new ways to meet the changing needs of students who were unable to attend on-campus classes. Nursing students have been taught by correspondence, telephone, video, CD-ROM, and Web-based learning. Much in the way that we as nurses have used our knowledge and strong assessment skills to diagnose and treat patients, we as nurse educators also continue to diagnose, assess, and develop innovative approaches to deliver excellent nursing education. We have customized that education based on our students' needs, available proven technology, and institutional resources. And equally important, we have maintained academic rigor.

Although nursing today remains rooted in traditional curriculum models, we are beginning to embrace new methods of curriculum design and delivery. Distance education is no longer only for those who are unable to get to campus but rather is offered, as a choice, for those who prefer it. As this modality gains momentum, we will continue to examine the characteristics of successful distance learners and evolve newer distance learning strategies. It is the online students of the last 10 years—true pioneers—who will develop and implement the evolving state of the art. In addition to learning from the learners, successful faculty will be studied and the teacher competencies required for distance education will be clarified, while barriers to, and incentives for, nursing faculty to teach via distance learning technology continue to be identified. Schools of nursing will take advantage of the practicality of sharing distance courses, become more flexible in transfer credit policies, and identify fairer ways to evaluate teacher effort and performance in distance learning when considering tenure and remuneration. The new "cybergogy" will encourage us to develop faculty sharing relationships among institutions of higher learning, and networks and consortia will be developed to make distance education possible for state, national, and international nursing use. Education will become more global and schools of nursing will utilize these consortia according to their individual needs. As dean of an online nursing program who has recruited a faculty made up of independent contractors from other institutions and educated them in online education, I am impressed by their teaching skills and talent, and especially by their dedication to our students scattered throughout the country. I am encouraged by watching them learn and implement technology while handling students who themselves are also learning this technology. With few exceptions, these educators came with little or no knowledge of online education. They were, however, experienced faculty, confident in their ability to teach nursing students and willing to learn a new teaching methodology. In doing so, they have demonstrated a level of professionalism that is both admirable and heartwarming. And after becoming familiar with the principles and best practices of distance education, they have brought these newly honed skills to their home schools and added distance learning to their traditional classrooms, thereby increasing the pool of nursing educators prepared in the pedagogy of distance education.

Distance education should not be considered a threat to traditional education, but rather an option in a list of ever-expanding choices that will encourage lifelong learning in the new millennium. The future of distance education and nursing is limitless and hard to imagine. I am confident, however, that we will do as we have done at each turning point in the past: continue to educate ourselves to meet the technological and societal challenges of the twenty-first century, maintain the rigor of the nursing curriculum, and continue to serve the needs of our students both near and far.

CHAPTER 1

An Overview
of Distance Education
and Web-Based Courses

Jeanne M. Novotny and Tami H. Wyatt

In a small town in rural Michigan, Jan, a 32-year-old advanced practice nurse and working mother, carries groceries from the car into her house. It is late afternoon and after putting the groceries away Jan sits down at her computer and logs in to a continuing education class. She takes a quiz to see if she got the main points of the last session. Jan then downloads a recommended reading that impacts the care she is delivering to one of her oncology patients. Next, she goes into a chat room and asks for specific information related to one of her patients from an expert and from other practitioners who are also enrolled in the same asynchronous continuing education program.

Tom, a 38-year-old registered nurse with an associate's degree, comes home from the evening shift at a large medical center in Atlanta. He has a midnight snack and logs on to his computer. Tom is taking a nursing theory class from a well-known professor. This class is one of the requirements for his baccalaureate degree. Tom accesses the library collection and downloads one of the required readings. A message comes across his computer screen from one of his classmates, who lives in Alaska. The

1

two communicate in their virtual chat space. Although they have never met face-to-face, they have become friends and plan to graduate at the same time.

These examples demonstrate how the Internet is revolutionizing nursing education. Jan and Tom have opportunities for continuous professional development because of the Internet and the distance education programs that are available. These are students who would not be found sitting in a traditional classroom. They are receiving a quality education that would be unavailable to them otherwise. Today, whether students enroll in a traditional learning experience or learn at a distance, the Internet will influence the way they learn because learning experiences are either Web-based, Web-enhanced, or Web-supported (Robley, Farnsworth, Flynn, & Horne, 2004). The purpose of this chapter is to review briefly the background of distance education, compare and contrast traditional and Internet instruction, and discuss the ways that the Internet is changing the classroom.

WHY DISTANCE EDUCATION?

Technology provides practicing nurses and nursing students with the opportunity to learn, share information, and collaborate with colleagues throughout the world. A distance education format will not meet the needs of all learners; however, it is ideal for the individual who is motivated, needs flexibility, and wants to maintain professional accountability through self-evaluation and ongoing education. Internet-based education is a learning option based on the assumption that students will become a part of a community of learners even as they work separately from each other and their instructors. Nurses not interested in using the Internet for educational purposes will also feel its effects because technology is changing the traditional classroom in subtle and profound ways.

Degree-granting institutions and continuing education programs are facing critical challenges. It is important to understand these challenges in order to understand why Internet education will become increasingly important in the twenty-first century. In order to remain viable, educational programs must do the following:

- Provide first-rate leadership and instruction in rapidly developing new areas of knowledge and specialization

- Meet the learning needs of an increasingly diverse student population

- Hire faculty that are flexible and have the ability to incorporate research findings and technology into everyday instructional practices

- Ensure quality learning standards and accreditation criteria that are comparable to face-to-face formats (Rosseter, 2003)

Because of these challenges, new ways of addressing the way we teach and how we learn are of the utmost importance. As universities, associations, private providers, and others compete in the marketplace for formal and continuing professional education, increasing numbers of learners will turn to the Internet as a convenient, satisfying, and economically prudent way to save time and money in order to keep current in their field. The Internet not only delivers online classes, but also creates "virtual communities" where professionals can communicate, get current information, and conduct business on a daily basis.

HISTORICAL PERSPECTIVE

Nurses have a rich history of seeking the latest method of getting the education they need to remain current. The evolution of American educational technology is slightly different from the technology used historically in nursing education. During the early 1900s, the American visual instruction movement and the radio movement established innovative forms of learning (Saettler, 1990), but it was not until the late twentieth century that the nursing profession began using film or video and radio technology as a form of distance education. The concept of using communication tools that are unbounded by time and space to bring education to learners far and wide began with print media and correspondence studies. This method required sending and receiving assignments via mail. The use of radio in education began as early as the 1920s and is still being used in developing countries. Only now, radio broadcasting for instructional purposes is computer-based radio (Nwaerondu & Thompson, 1999). By World War II, educators in the United States were more interested in television technology. Television technology became popular in the 1960s when a variety of video-based initiative television systems became available. This form of broadcast uses asynchronous transfer mode (ATM) via videoconferencing equipment. Typically, programs use ATM videoconferencing equipment with televisions, connecting two or more classrooms to one another with an instructor in one of the locations. This technology is still used today because of its close resemblance to the traditional classroom but this costly method is gradually being replaced with other technology-rich methods of instruction (Reiser, 2001). Some nursing programs combine various forms of distance education modalities to attract students in far-off places. These programs, known as external degree programs, use video or film technology, print media, videoconferencing technology, and the Internet to deliver instruction. They differ from traditional programs because the learning experience does not offer a prescribed method of learning. The learning is not merely a transfer of material from the classroom to the Internet. Instead distance education uses different methods of delivery, reinforcement, and communication with classmates and the teacher; and the learning is independent (Hyde & Murray, 2005).

Computer technology for distance education has leaped to the forefront partly because of technological advances and educational reform as well (Armstrong, Gessner, & Cooper, 2000). According to the 2001 National Survey of Information Technology in U.S. Higher Education, 56% of college and universities offer full online courses (Escoffery, Miner, & Alperin, 2003). This statistic does not include colleges or universities that offer portions of a course online. The Internet is the most versatile distance education vehicle of the information age, with users becoming information seekers. In fact, because of the Internet and the information age, learners are bombarded with information and must evaluate the validity of the information. This was not necessarily the case prior to the information age. Information was limited and required extensive seeking and research skills to obtain little information. Because of the Internet and advancing technology, all aspects of nursing will be affected, including opportunities and approaches to learning.

The need for degree completion, skill acquisition, continuing education, and certificate nursing education will continue to proliferate. A shift in restructured health care environments to an emphasis on primary and ambulatory care provided in clinics, community, and other settings, requires additional knowledge, skills, and expertise. Nurses seeking to remain competitive in the health care market will need the community assessment, problem-solving, and clinical management skills that are taught at the baccalaureate level (Beason, 1997). Historically, nursing always has been able to evolve continuously in its methods, structure, and educational approaches to meet the changing health care needs of society. Distance education can meet the health care challenges of society and the profession in a way that is both clinically relevant and educationally viable because distance education can be delivered through Web-based technologies, interactive videoconferencing via Internet, and pre-recorded media (Dudding & Purcell-Robertson, 2003).

DIFFERENCES BETWEEN TRADITIONAL AND INTERNET INSTRUCTION

Distance education is defined as planned learning that occurs in a different place from teaching, requiring interactive technology in real time or delayed, and a course design supportive of distance education (Escoffery et al., 2003). The two basic models of distance education are synchronous and asynchronous modes of interactivity (Table 1.1). In synchronous learning, the teacher and the student interact in real time, similar to traditional classroom settings, but this method decreases flexibility. It requires all students to be online, in a videoconference, or in a virtual classroom at the same time. Asynchronous learning occurs when individuals access the educational materials independently and at times and places of their choice. Asynchronous activities allow students to take as much time as they want to read the materials and compose responses or messages. It also allows time for reflection and may result in thoughtful discussion. The use of asynchronous technology extends the reach of education to previously underserved populations as well as to those who prefer a more self-directed learning environment (Lewis, 2000). It is the most flexible and friendly way to use the Internet for formal degree programs and continuing education.

Distance learning offers new opportunities for nurses who are seeking basic or advanced degrees, certificates, or lifelong learning for professional development (Billings et al., 2001). The advantages to using the Internet are many. First, convenience and easy access are the cornerstones. The course work may be self-paced and asynchronous, and the student has easy access to online libraries, databases, and learning resources. The ability to network with colleagues in specialty areas without any geographic limitations is unlimited. There are several disadvantages. First, the student needs a computer, modem, Internet service provider, and basic computer literacy skills (Novotny & Murley, 1999). Second, bandwidth and connectivity to the Internet are issues that continue to exist in Internet-based education. This is especially true for individuals who rely on modems to connect to the Internet versus students with broad-bandwidth connections (i.e., DSL, cable, satellite). Third, individual learners must recognize their personal learning style and determine if Internet-based education is appropriate. The work in developing and implementing a quality distance education program occurs before students ever begin. The spirit and potential of distance education can best be realized by programs that are specifically designed and implemented on the basis of the needs of the identified population of learners for whom the program is intended.

TABLE 1.1　Asynchronous Versus Synchronous Distance Learning Methodologies Via the Internet

Learning Methodology	Asynchronous	Synchronous
Video	Prerecorded Webcasts, videoconference, or presentation to be viewed at student's convenience	Real-time videoconference streaming: One-way videoconferencing: learner can see and hear the conference but cannot interact with the speaker. Two-way videoconferencing: learner can see, hear, and interact with the speaker by typing responses, or by voice and video with videoconferencing technology
Document Sharing/ Assignments	Sending documents or assignments via e-mail, listservs, or threaded discussion or storing documents on Web page	Sharing of documents using courseware management systems, or other applications that allow real-time document sharing
Discussion	Listservs, threaded discussions, newsgroups, e-mail	Chat rooms, real-time videoconferencing
Presentations	Multimedia or electronic presentations, case study, video tutorials, Webcasts, text-based tutorials, interactive tutorials	Real-time videoconference streaming, audio/ document sharing
Evaluation	Online surveys, tests, threaded discussions, newsgroups, listservs, document sharing of assignments via e-mail	Real-time document/ audio sharing, videoconference streaming

The advantages of a distance education program are

- Individualized pacing with active student involvement
- Instructional assistance during and outside of regular class times
- Multiple media formats resulting in greater interactivity
- On-time assessment, feedback, and reinforcement
- Individualized and collaborative learning
- Optimal use of instructor's expertise
- Information linked to student pace and performance

Understanding the differences between traditional learning and Internet learning is essential before undertaking an online program of any kind because students and educators who embark on a distance education program must change their thinking about how they learn or teach. Regardless of the technology used, certain instructional functions must exist (Heinich, Molenda, Russell, & Smaldino, 1999):

- Instructor presentation of content using multimedia-rich technology with supporting printed material
- Student-teacher interaction such as discussion, assignments, or testing
- Student-student interaction in small groups, pairs, threaded discussions, or group projects

IMPORTANT THEMES

There are several themes that shape online education and the future direction of learning and teaching. These themes, developed by Kearsley (2000), are all interrelated and overlapping but are important for the potential student.

1. *Collaboration:* The single biggest change that the Internet brings to education is the increased collaboration between students and teachers, which includes diverse individuals in all parts of the world. Many activities and projects involve information-sharing activities. Even when there is not specific intent to collaborate, it often happens anyway because it is so easy to interact online.

2. *Connectivity:* These activities include discussion boards, chat rooms, e-mail, conferences, and group projects. Students and instructors can easily connect across time and geographic location. Another important aspect of connectivity in nursing education is that students can interact directly with experts in their field of study. This is especially important in advanced nursing practice where current protocols frequently reside on the Internet. Efficient connectivity and response times are crucial for effective learning. There are three important limits to consider with respect to response times and connectivity: (a) a learner feels connected if he or she is able to retrieve information or access a page within one tenth of a second; (b) a learner's flow of thought will be interrupted if connection takes more than 1 second; (c) a learner will stay focused on a text-based dialogue only if the interruptions between the discussion are less than 10 seconds (Nielsen, 2001).

3. *Student-centered:* When experienced nurses return to school for further formal education, they respond well to a program that is based on adult learning principles. These principles, developed by Malcolm Knowles (1980), are based on the assumption that the student is a capable decision-maker and is an active participant rather than a passive receiver in the teaching-learning process. Teachers must recognize the value of a less hierarchical learning environment and embrace the role of facilitator as their primary function. One of the most important contributions of this work is to increase awareness of the learner's rightful place at the center of the instructional process.

4. *Unbounded:* The Internet offers online education that eliminates the walls of the classroom. It gives students access to information and people anywhere in the world. Online education removes boundaries having to do with where and when students learn as well as who can be a learner. This is especially important for continuing education for professional nurses.

5. *Virtual Community:* A sense of community is important, whether it is the community of learners defined by a particular school or continuing education program or a physical community such as a town or city. The Internet makes it possible to define virtual communities around common interests and work-related activities. A community is only possible if a sense of presence is created. Audio and sound are important in creating presence.

6. *Exploration:* The Internet allows learners to integrate knowledge into their own behavior and belief system and to create new knowledge and insight that can only come when there is the

adventure of discovery. Many online activities involve adventure or discovery learning. Problem-based learning is an example of this type of learning activity.

7. *Shared Knowledge:* Nursing professionals and students can tap into a vast knowledge network and they can contribute as well. Information on the Internet is immediately available to anyone in the world at any time. Sharing knowledge is the core of education but prior to computer networks this was only accomplished in limited ways.

8. *Multisensory Experience:* Learning theories tell us that learning is more effective when it involves multiple sensory channels such as visuals, color, movement, sound, voice, touch, and smell. For example, Edgar Dale's classic cone of experience theory suggests that individuals learn approximately 10% of read material, 50% of observed demonstrations and material read, and 80% of material that is interactive (Dale, 1969). Multimedia technology is available on the Internet and can provide most kinds of learning experiences except for touch and smell. Although these experiences may not be perfect, they are often much better than traditional learning activities that are primarily based on lectures.

9. *Authenticity:* Internet education is highly authentic in nature. Students can access actual databases and experts. This gives the educational experience relevance to the learning needs of the student. The Internet provides direct access to major repositories of research information, a critical component of nursing.

Since distance education methods penetrated nursing education in the 1990s, there has been ample research examining these themes. Overwhelmingly, distance education experiences that promote community building and interactivity among the students and with the instructor are key elements to more positive student experiences with greater perceived learning opportunities (Hyde & Murray, 2005; Robley et al., 2004).

WHAT TO EXPECT WITH ONLINE LEARNING OR TRADITIONAL CLASSES CONNECTED TO THE INTERNET

Until now, the primary function of a teacher has been to transfer knowledge, with the student in a passive role. A majority of teaching and learning is passive and most students find this style of learning very safe and comfortable. Distance education students and teachers need to be prepared for a change in this approach. When the Internet becomes the primary vehicle for learners to receive information and skills, classes that primarily transfer information become obsolete. Instead the student becomes an active participant in the process. The role of the instructor is to make the information meaningful, create a positive learning environment, integrate knowledge into the learner's own belief system, and create new knowledge and insight that come only when three or more learners are engaged in intense discussion and exploration.

In some programs, clinical skills are evaluated by connecting students to instructors, using portable videoconferencing devices such as Webcam technology with two-way videoconferencing. Firefighters, pilots, and even nurses are learning skills through simulated virtual-reality videos and manikins. Those teaching in online learning environments must be prepared to deliver instruction with various online learning modalities in order to meet the diverse learning styles of individuals, similar to the preparations that are adopted in the traditional classroom setting for students with various learning styles. Teachers and students must also be prepared to create a "community" of learners by encouraging discussion, participation, and presence that may require the use of more advanced technology such as audio capability.

Technology and the Internet specifically are changing the way individuals learn and gather data. Nursing students are using more Internet resources to support clinical decisions, access information, and plan care. Furthermore, teachers are using the Internet in traditional classroom settings to access information, demonstrate processes or mechanisms (i.e., animated blood flow through the heart), and promote in-class small-group learning activities with wireless mobile technology. Tablet PCs with handwriting-recognition features and personal digital assistants are used in many progressive classroom settings. Students may access drug databases electronically during lectures or use medical calculators for more complex algorithms while learning fluid and electrolyte disturbances in the patient who is immunosuppressed.

In conclusion, the academic quality and legitimacy of well-designed and well-executed distance education programs have been proved (Lewis, 2000). Don't be afraid to reach out and teach or enroll in a distance education course. In fact, if you plan to teach an online course, become an online course learner first. You will be embracing an important skill that will prepare you for nursing practice in the twenty-first century.

REFERENCES

Armstrong, M. L., Gessner, B. A., & Cooper, S. S. (2000). Pots, pans, and the pearls: The nursing profession's rich history with distance education for a new century of nursing. *Journal of Continuing Education in Nursing, 31*(2), 63–70.

Beason, C. F. (1997). Distance learning—Education to prepare nurses for practice in the 21st century. In V. Ferguson (Ed.), *Educating the 21st century nurse: Challenges and opportunities.* New York: NLN Press.

Billings, D. M., Ward, J. W., & Penton-Cooper, L. (2001). Distance learning in nursing. *Seminars in Oncology Nursing, 17*(1), 48–54.

Dale, E. (1969). *Audiovisual methods in teaching* (3rd ed.). New York: Holt, Rinehart & Winston.

Dudding, C. C., & Purcell-Robertson, R. M. (2003). Beyond the technology. *ASHA Leader, 6*(10), 6–7, 16.

Escoffery, C., Miner, K. R., & Alperin, M. (2003). Ten informative Web sites on distance education. *American Journal of Health Behavior, 27,* 464–465.

Heinich, R., Molenda, M., Russell, J. D., & Smaldino, S. E. (1999). *Instructional media and technologies for learning.* Upper Saddle River, NJ: Simon & Schuster.

Hyde, A., & Murray, M. (2005). Nurses' experiences of distance education programmes. *Journal of Advanced Nursing, 49*(1), 87–95.

Kearsley, G. (2000). *Online education: Learning and teaching in cyberspace.* Belmont, CA: Wadsworth/Thomson Learning.

Knowles, M. S. (1980). *The modern practice of adult education: From pedagogy to androgogy.* Chicago: Follett.

Lewis, J. M. (2000). Distance education foundations. In J. M. Novotny (Ed.), *Distance education in nursing* (pp. 4–22). New York: Springer.

Nielsen, J. (2001). Jakob Nielsen on e-learning. Retrieved March 13, 2005, from http://www.elearningpost.com/features/archives/001015.asp

Novotny, J. M., & Murley, J. (1999). Designing successful learning programs. *Nursing Leadership Forum, 4*(1), 10–13.

Nwaerondu, N. G., & Thompson, G. (1999). The use of educational radio in developing countries: Lessons from the past. Retrieved March 13, 2005, from http://www1.worldbank.org/disted/Technology/broadcast/rad-01.html

Reiser, R. A. (2001). A history of instructional design and technology. *Educational Technology Research and Development, 49*(2), 57–67.

Robley, L. R., Farnsworth, B. J., Flynn, J. B., & Horne, C. D. (2004). This new house: Building knowledge through online learning. *Journal of Professional Nursing, 20,* 333–342.

Rosseter, R. (2003). Alliance for nursing accreditation releases new statement on distance education policies. *Nursing News, 27*(3), 29.

Saettler, P. (1990). *The evolution of American education technology.* Englewood, CA: Libraries Unlimited.

PART 1

Teaching and Learning Strategies for Distance Education

CHAPTER 2

Teaching a Web-Based Course: Lessons from the Front

Mary L. McHugh

The types of people who need educational services from colleges and universities—and especially the ways in which they need those services delivered—have changed over time. Therefore, the people who teach in colleges and universities must adjust their skills to meet the needs of the students they will be serving in the twenty-first century. The focus of this chapter is on the skills and techniques needed for teaching Web-based courses.

College students of the 1950s and 1960s expected that what they learned in their college education classes would last most of their careers. Of course, they would expect to update knowledge, but at a fairly slow and steady pace, and much of what they learned would remain valid for most of their careers. Instead, knowledge longevity has proven far shorter than expected and is becoming ever shorter. For example, the overall pool of scientific knowledge doubles every 19 months (Sparrow, 2004). Children of the Baby Boomer generation have gone back to college in the 1990s and 2000s just to be able to hold on to their jobs (Heinke & Russum, 2001). Their younger colleagues of Generation X, the Y-generation, and the Nexers must expect to renew their knowledge completely every 5 years and to update knowledge constantly immediately upon graduation.

These changes in knowledge requirements mean that as college and university teachers, we no longer should expect to educate degree-bound classes and then say good-bye forever, except for reunions and the occasional greeting card from our students. Rather, the model is going to be that we will need to maintain two educational tracks for students in our schools: the degree track and the continuing education track. And in both tracks, the convenience of Web-based education is going to be in high demand.

In the very recent past and even today, some teachers have been and are able to refuse to learn to teach online. It is the opinion of this author that this stance is unwise in the extreme. Even today, I hear from many new graduates of doctoral programs that part of their interview for new faculty positions includes the questions, "Are you able and willing to teach online courses?" And it is made very clear to them that if the answer is no, the position will not be open to them. I predict that by the year 2010, in those colleges and universities that have a significant Web course presence, all faculty will be required to accept both online and on-campus course assignments as part of their employment contract. In fact, it may be that in the future, schools will be more tolerant of faculty who are able to teach online but not able to teach in the classroom. For example, in order to facilitate diversity, they may be able to hire foreign-born teachers whose spoken English language skills would be problematic for classroom lectures but would pose no problem for online courses. Thus, in some schools, some teachers may be employed to teach exclusively online courses. And while there will continue to be a steady demand for classroom classes, the demand for online courses will continue to increase exponentially.

The reason for the demand in online courses is that the proportion of students who are able to live on or near campus and attend school full-time is continually decreasing. Both matriculated, degree-bound students and continuing education students are less likely to be able to go to school full time than was the case in the 1970s and 1980s. Beginning with the 1980s, we saw a trend for even degree-bound students to be independent adults, and in many cases, to be older (in their 30s and above) with families and full-time jobs. Of course, this is typical of continuing education students. For these students, it is very difficult to travel to the school at a specific class time, to find parking, and to attend class.

For many, perhaps even the majority of continuing education students, Web-based courses are their only option for updating their certified educational knowledge base and expanding their certified professional skills. Of course, people can always update their knowledge informally. But increasingly, professionals are required to prove through transcripts, Continuing Education credits, and other formal certification methods to show proof of their updated professional knowledge and skills. Many professional nurses are turning to colleges and universities for academic courses for this type of continuing education and they need to access this education via Web-based courses.

This chapter is written for those members of university instructional communities who are interested in focusing more energy in teaching online courses through the Internet. It will address the differences among traditional, correspondence, and Web-based modalities for teaching undergraduate and graduate courses. Strengths and limitations of each modality will be addressed. Techniques of developing and implementing a Web-based course and degrees through the Web will be discussed, with special emphasis on how to adapt teaching methods to the Internet. Techniques that have proved unsuccessful will be presented, as well as tips for success.

KEY DEFINITIONS: THE NATURE OF THE BEAST

A *traditional on-campus course,* also called a "classroom course," is defined as a course in which students attend class in a college or university classroom one or more times per week, purchase their text materials at the university bookstore, and receive paper handouts in class from the instructor. Study guides may be purchased or made available in learning labs on campus. The student-instructor interaction is either face-to-face or via telephone. Often, students have group projects for which they schedule themselves during their out-of-class time. Students have access to the books, journals, and other materials in the on-campus library and for a fee can obtain other materials through interlibrary loan. Traditionally, on-campus courses make the assumption that some students may not have access to the Internet, and the course can be successfully completed without that access.

A *correspondence course* is defined as a course in which there is no on-campus requirement. The student pays a single fee for tuition, books, and supportive materials. Usually, the student must independently study the materials, schedule exams, and mail the exams back to the college or university for grading. When the student completes all requirements, a grade is sent. That is, there may or may not be any provision for communication between students and faculty, such as through mail or telephone calls. Typically, there is a final deadline for completion of all requirements, but the deadline is usually generous and students may learn at their own pace.

A *Web-supported course* is a traditional on-campus course in which students have access to all the resources listed above. In addition, the course instructor places some materials on the Internet for students to use and perhaps copy if they wish. Such materials as the course syllabus, study guides, assignment guides, grading criteria, lecture notes, and slide presentations from the class lectures may be made available to students at the class Internet site. A Web-supported course may or may not *require* students to use the Internet. For those who have no personal access, the instructor may provide the materials through class, library, or lab. The university may provide access through student computer labs or in student dormitories. Access to the course Internet site may be open or password-protected. Typically, a Web-supported course will offer an online discussion board or chat room to enhance class discussions. In addition to traditional student-faculty interactions, a Web-supported course usually makes a faculty e-mail address available to students for additional interaction opportunities. Students also may have special group "meetings" via computer conferencing technology. Both real-time and virtual meetings can be supported in the Internet environment. Also, students can obtain more information about course topics through either personal or faculty-guided Web searches. The two key criteria for a Web-supported course are that (1) an on-campus classroom component is required, and (2) at least some of the course materials are available on the Web (although the course may permit students to obtain all their materials without accessing the Web).

A *blended* course is a course that has both on-campus classroom and Web-course requirements. Typically, these courses have one or more intensive on-campus class days followed by some weeks or months of Web-course work. Some teachers feel that these types of courses overcome the limitations of a Web course (loss of the face-to-face meetings between instructor and student, and loss of demonstrations that teachers believe can be done only in person), but allow people to be distance students because they require only a few days of on-campus work. Many college faculty are of the opinion that people who "really want the education" can afford and arrange to get to campus for the few days or so of intensive on campus instruction that blended courses require. In my experience, that is not the case. Many students will choose another program if a program has too many intensives, and some will not come if there are any intensives. Intensives are most useful to students who have sufficient control over their work schedule that they can take vacation days for the intensive classes, or who live near enough campus that they can travel to the classes, or who have the economic resources to fly to campus and pay for hotel and per diem expenses necessary to stay in the city where the campus is located for the intensive on-campus classes. That excludes quite a lot of students.

A *Web-based course* is one in which the entire course is online. This modality requires that all students have access to the Internet. The syllabus, including course description, objectives, class schedule (if any), handouts, examinations, class discussions, and so on are all available only through the Internet. Some of these courses require the student to purchase a computer video camera and have software that can send, receive, and play the streaming video along with the video camera. This allows the students to give oral presentations in the class, and to receive videotaped learning materials and to handle all sorts of video learning media. Texts and other required materials that must be purchased are available by mail from the university bookstore. Students typically communicate with each other and the faculty via a combination of discussion board, chat room, and e-mail. Faculty may or may not provide lecture materials to support required readings. Typically, faculty provide information about important links to relevant sites on the Web, but students are also expected to do considerable work in personal searches to enhance their own learning.[1] A Web-based course may or may not adhere to the traditional semester or quarter schedule of the university in which it is housed. Web courses, like correspondence courses, may permit the student wide latitude about scheduling readings, homework, projects, and examinations. The three key criteria for a Web-based course are as follows:

1. There is no on-campus requirement for any part of the course. This means that everything—from registration, enrollment, and payment of tuition and fees to content presentations and group projects—can be handled through the Internet or via e-mail or the U.S. mail system. Thus, students who live in the same city as the university have no advantage over students who live halfway around the world.

2. All of the required course materials are either available online or may be purchased via mail order from the university bookstore or another mail-order supplier such as Amazon.com, Barnes andnoble.com, or any other online bookstore.

3. Students who live a great distance from each other and from the faculty can communicate with faculty and other students via e-mail and perhaps through some combination of discussion boards, computer conferencing, or chat rooms, although phone calls may be used occasionally.

ADVANTAGES AND LIMITATIONS
OF EDUCATIONAL MODALITIES

Traditional On-Campus Courses

Traditional on-campus courses offer many advantages. The format is familiar to students who have attended high school. The daily or weekly class schedule and deadlines for papers, projects, and exams provide a form of external discipline. The instructor and student have the advantage of face-to-face discussions. This is perhaps the greatest advantage the traditional classroom format can offer. Students and faculty mutually benefit from vigorous, in-person, intellectual discussions about the content of the course. When students and faculty discuss problems, identify potential solutions, and hear each others' ideas, a great deal of learning can take place. All can hear the words, inflections, and feeling tone of each others' utterances and at the same time gain further information from the body language of both the speaker and the listeners. Of course, the teacher ensures that content is current and can offer personal support to the student who struggles with some of the content. This modality has been in use for as long as formal education has existed because it is so successful for most people.

    This format does create some problems. First, the student must arrange his or her schedule to fit the scheduled time of the course. This requirement may exclude many people from the class, simply due to scheduling problems. Second, for many students, travel to and from the university and parking are significant problems. For some adult students, class attendance can require a 2- or 3-hour drive. Although most graduate classes meet only once a week for 3 hours, adding in the drive time means that students must allocate 7 to 9 hours per week just for class attendance. Homework, study, and library time require another 9 hours. Parking at our university is a problem. Most universities were built for use by young (17- to 22-year-olds), physically healthy students who live on campus in dormitories or less than 10 blocks away in student housing. These students walk to classes, libraries, and university activities. Almost none of our graduate students and fewer than half of our undergraduate students fit this profile today. For some people, physical disabilities are such that attendance at a traditional classroom course is difficult. Third, although this format allows for in-class discussion, those discussions must be very limited in time. Classrooms are often in demand, and the students and instructor must vacate in time for the next class to begin. Fourth, shy students are at a great disadvantage. Particularly in large classes, only brave or aggressive students may get the chance to ask their questions or offer their opinions. In fact, in classes with more than 12–15 students, somebody will almost always be overlooked. In my classes that have more than 20 students, I estimate that only about 50% to 75% of the students *ever* speak in class and only 10% regularly contribute. Many of the others are too shy to speak in class.

Although people seldom talk about drop-out rates with traditional classroom courses, attrition is a problem that nobody quite knows how to measure. Some people do not count as attrition those who register but drop a course during the regular drop/add period; they only count as attrition those who drop the course after that period. Others believe that attrition should include all those who drop a course after registering for the course as do distance education programs. Because of the difference in measurement methods, it is impossible to compare directly attrition rates between traditional classroom courses and distance education courses at this time. However, most researchers claim that traditional classroom education has the lowest attrition rates of all the modalities (Parker, 1999; Phipps & Merisotis, 1999; Thompson, 1997). Drop-out rates for traditional classroom courses vary greatly (depending upon program and whether the student is in a degree-bound program or in continuing education) but range from as low as zero to as high as 40%.

Correspondence Courses

Correspondence courses have long offered an educational opportunity to people whose location or job made traditional classroom education impossible. They have also been an important resource to people whose physical disabilities make it impossible to attend a regular classroom. Many people living in areas far from colleges and universities do not have the money to give up work and move to a college location. Some people are employed in jobs that require a great deal of travel; others are required to work rotating shifts; still others live too far from a college or for other reasons are unable to meet the requirements of a traditional classroom schedule. In the past, correspondence courses offered one of the few options for college credit to all these people. Most correspondence courses provide generous deadlines for course completion. For people who learn in ways different from those of typical students and who therefore cannot succeed in a traditional classroom, correspondence courses may facilitate learning success by allowing the student to take all the time needed to learn and may give students more latitude to use personally developed learning techniques.

The correspondence course format does have some drawbacks. First, by its nature, it offers limited faculty support. This is a barrier to students when their reading materials are insufficient or when the student's work processes are ineffective. Second, for many students, the student-to-student interaction can facilitate great learning and unfortunately, there is little to no student cohort support available in a correspondence course format. Third, correspondence courses may not work well for highly changeable content. The materials must be prepared months or even years in advance, and updates may be difficult to incorporate into the course. For some types of courses, such as computing, advertising, and medical topics, changes in the field may occur so rapidly that the correspondence course format simply cannot keep up. Fourth, correspondence courses have a much higher reported noncompletion rate than the other formats presented in this chapter. The attrition (noncompletion) rate of correspondence courses is as high as 80% in some reports (Heinke & Russum, 2001). This is probably a function of all of the above factors. It may also be due to the lack of human contact. The act of communicating with a teacher on a regular basis can serve as a strong impetus to study and complete assignments so as to avoid losing face.

Web-Supported Courses

Web-supported courses are essentially enhanced traditional courses. They have generally the same advantages and disadvantages as traditional courses. The Web is used as an additional learning opportunity and may greatly increase communication among faculty and students. It also may ease some of the problems of obtaining syllabi, class handouts, and other paper materials because most universities increasingly restrict copying expenses. It is also cheaper for the student to download these materials than to have to purchase them from the campus bookstore or copying center. Web-support courses may greatly enhance the value of the course to shy students who are unlikely to speak up in class.

If the Web supports include e-mail to faculty and other students or chat room or discussion board facilities, the student's shyness may cease to be a problem. Shyness is generally a reticence in the physical presence of others. However, most shy people feel quite comfortable with computer communications. The only disadvantage of these courses is for the few students who have no Internet access and for those who may be resistant to using computers. This is a vanishing problem as time passes, but may still be a problem for a very small number of students.

Attrition rates in these courses have not been specifically addressed in the literature. Presumably, students with no Internet access either will not sign up for these courses or will obtain Internet materials from the instructor or another student. However, because these courses are essentially traditional classroom courses with a bit of Internet support—often optional—they probably have the same drop-out rates as any other classroom course.

Blended Courses

Blended courses attempt to offer all the advantages of both traditional classroom and Internet courses. They can be extremely costly for some students because they require distance students to travel to the location of the school for the intensive classes, assuming that the classroom portion of the course is offered in an intensive format. (By "intensive" is meant that the student spends one to five consecutive intensive class days in the classroom. If the classroom portion is offered throughout the semester, the course is considered Internet-supported rather than a blended course.) For many students, that travel is accompanied by the need for temporary lodging, meals, and perhaps parking expenses, in addition to the tuition and travel expenses.

For the kind of courses the author of this chapter teaches, those travel and lodging expenses, added to tuition expense, are impossible for approximately 90% to 98% of the students. However, this format can be extremely valuable for certain types of courses. It is especially useful for nursing courses with an assessment or skills learning component that can be taught in an intensive format. Then the remainder of the theory material can be taught online for the rest of the semester. It permits students to obtain new hands-on skills in a clinical technology lab in the intensive format, and then to go back home and perhaps work with a preceptor in their home community to practice and hone those skills in a home-based clinical. At the same time, the student can continue to learn more in-depth clinical theory to support the assessment skills.

Sometimes, however, the blended format is used because the teacher is not yet comfortable with online teaching. Some teachers subject their students to the expense and inconvenience of travel, lodging, and meals simply because the teacher has decided that no distance course allows the "quality" that can be delivered in a face-to-face format. Such teachers either do not know or have no faith in the research that shows no differences in learning performance between traditional classroom courses and distance education courses for most subjects (Russell, 1998; Zolkos, 1999). In such cases, it is suggested that colleges and universities that allow teachers to force students to travel and incur lodging and meal expenses for unnecessary intensives will soon find demand for their courses declining. Distance students will find plentiful options at schools that recognize blended courses should be reserved for those very few subjects absolutely requiring hands-on teaching experiences. Such courses include content such as dissection in biology class, suturing and casting in the emergency care class, and other such skills content.

Web-Based Courses

This relatively new modality offers nothing essentially new to the educational process, yet properly handled may combine advantages of several of the other modalities. As with traditional on-campus courses, personal communications among teachers and students are a great strength of the format. Although contact is remote, it can (and should) be frequent. The best Internet teachers plan to answer e-mail from students daily or at least two to three times per week. Students often form online study and project groups, and those students will often communicate with each other several times a day. The students may lose some communicative power because of the loss of physical or visual contact during communication. However, that may not be much of a factor as students become more accustomed to the Internet.

Even though people are not physically together at all and may not even be together simultaneously, they are still able to communicate effectively if they have any degree of comfort with computers. More and more people have grown accustomed to personal and business use of e-mail, chat rooms, and discussion boards. Many believe they are able to communicate *better* through the computer than in person. They believe there is less miscommunication because the written word can be viewed and edited prior to sending it, and inadvertent negative voice tones can be edited out. One is less likely to blurt out something untoward when the communication is written. Also, nobody is ever interrupted.

One great advantage of Web courses is their effect on people who have physical (speech or hearing) disabilities, accents, or who are just quiet or shy by nature. None of these characteristics has anything to do with intelligence, creativity, or potential class contributions. However, these kinds of barriers can seriously interfere with a student's ability or willingness to participate as a full member of the class. Unfortunately, human prejudice being what it is, class members also may misinterpret another's disability as a lack of intelligence. Essentially, the Web wipes out the effects of all of these problems.

As previously mentioned, shyness and most physical disabilities are not factors in writing or computer communications. People who are typically quiet in a group often find much to communicate via the computer. Shyness (and quietness may be a form of shyness) is typically a reaction to the physical presence in one location of many strangers or casual acquaintances. Students in our Internet classes have often told us they have never before felt so comfortable participating fully in a class. They are amazed and delighted that shyness is simply not a factor in Internet courses. As teachers, we find this a truly delightful effect. The input of people with a history of withholding their comments in class because of disabilities of one kind or another often proves to be astute, interesting, and highly stimulating to the entire class.

Other advantages include the ability of students to do class work at their own convenience. Students whose jobs require a lot of travel can take along a portable computer or use an Internet café. Students can do class work anywhere and anytime. If traveling students are in a location where there is no local Internet service, good organization can work to keep long-distance calls to their own ISP very short. The student can call in and download lectures and discussion items to the hard drive and then sign off the Internet. The student can then study the materials on the laptop computer. Students should always use a word processor to construct their papers anyway. E-mail items and discussion board items also can be constructed locally on a word processor. Then, with a short second long-distance call to the ISP, the student simply uses the cut-and-paste function to move communications from local programs to the course Internet site. Costly calls might be occasioned only if a student wishes to do a lengthy search on the Internet for further information on a class topic. However, many students will organize their time in such a way that those searches are scheduled when they have access to a local Internet service.

The final advantage of Web-based courses is that they satisfy customer demand. More and more people are asking that courses and whole degree programs be offered online. They are extremely convenient in terms of time for students who live busy lives and who have great difficulty with scheduling. Nurses may have to work different shifts, so scheduling 3 or 4 hours a week in class at the same time every week for 15 weeks may be impossible. Faculty sometimes do not realize how inconvenient getting to class can be, especially for older students who may be dealing with arthritis, nurses with back pain, and people who live a long way from the school. Driving time to the school can be significant for some people and add as much as 3 to 4 hours to the amount of time spent in class. Then students still have to find parking, and parking can be a serious difficulty at many universities. There may be parking expenses. Parking may be located some blocks from the classroom and walking several blocks, especially in bad weather, for a 50-year-old student can be a significant deterrence to attending classes. And remember, these older students are also trying to maintain demanding full-time jobs and participate in family life. Their time is at a premium and all these factors make an online course extremely attractive. The convenience factor is becoming increasingly critical to many adult students and outweighs the disadvantages listed below. Student demand for online courses may force some colleges and universities to choose between offering more of their courses online or downsizing to fit the reduced number of traditional, full-time, on-campus students.

Web-based courses do have some disadvantages. Eight key disadvantages are presented here: First, *the student must have access to a computer and an Internet link. Not everybody has this technology in the home or office.* If students have to come to campus anyway to use computer labs, several of the key advantages of an online course are lost. Second, *some students are still not computer-literate; for them this modality may be ineffective.* However, this disadvantage is rapidly declining as more people worldwide become very Internet-literate. During the next 10 years, virtually all undergraduate college students will have grown up using computers and the Internet in school. Most prospective graduate students will come to school already using the Internet in their personal lives. They will feel as comfortable with Internet communications as they do with physical-presence communication.

Third, *although the Internet is quite adaptable to most theory courses, there remain many challenges to teaching hands-on skills content through this medium.* Even more important is the need to personally watch students perform certain types of tasks if their skill level is to be assessed. For example, there have been many films developed for medical and nursing students on how to start an intravenous (IV) infusion. However, watching a film will not produce a competent practitioner. The students typically practice on an artificial arm model before attempting to start an IV on a patient. Much development on how to use the Internet to teach and evaluate skill tasks remains to be done before certain kinds of courses can be offered entirely online. One way this problem can be addressed is to reduce rather than eliminate on-campus course work. At the University of Colorado at Denver and Health Sciences Center School of Nursing, we are making increased use of blended courses and courses that are taught entirely in an intensive on-campus format for hands-on skills content and offering students the option to take their theory courses online.

Fourth, *many teachers are not yet sufficiently familiar with this format as an educational tool to function as instructors of Internet courses.* Some are highly resistant to learning to teach on the Internet. Access to education on Internet teaching is now widely available to nursing faculty through the National League for Nursing (NLN) and through the University of Indiana. However, resistance to learning to teach in this modality dies hard for some teachers. And it is not correct to say that the impending retirement of older teachers will solve the problem. Some of the people who were most eager to learn to teach on the Internet were older members of the faculty and some of the most resistant have been some of the younger members of the faculty. These problems will probably be solved over time as teaching Internet courses is made a requirement of employment, but in the early 2000s this is still a significant barrier to the development of online course offerings in many schools.

Fifth, *some teachers continue to be extremely concerned about the possible loss of learning of certain types of content due to the loss of face-to-face class discussions.* Personally, we do not give this argument much credence. The evidence to date shows that learning for Internet courses equals and sometimes even exceeds learning in the traditional classroom format. However, the political fallout from the argument about the credibility of online courses is a great disadvantage at this time. Many members of university faculties are extremely skeptical of using the Internet to offer courses. They refuse to prepare their courses for the online format and politick against their departments and universities moving in this direction. We suspect much of this resistance is occasioned more by a personal fear of having to change their teaching approach than by an honest consideration of evidence of learning in Internet courses. The many concerns about lower learning for students in online courses have not been validated, and personal experience has shown this author that learning levels in both modalities are highly dependent upon student commitment to learning. In fact, some people who are very popular classroom teachers may not be able to adapt to the new format. Some experts can, with very little preparation time, simply enter the classroom and give a fine lecture. This approach is not appropriate for the Internet. Thus, for at least some faculty, Internet courses will require much more work than traditional classroom courses.

Sixth, *this modality is still so new that the infrastructure to support Web-based courses is still inadequate in many colleges.* A good Internet education program requires the school to hire or dedicate media resources people to support the software and infrastructure. Even with this support, teachers may have to spend a great deal of time at the beginning of the semester helping their students get registered with the university and enrolled in the course, obtaining course passwords, and making sure that students are able to work with the technology used in the course. In a traditional course, the admissions office, the registrar's office, the bookstore, and sometimes lab assistants handle these kinds of things. Typically, online course faculty are not paid more for this extra work and are not given higher workload credit for teaching an online course. Thus, this work may not be counted in the teacher's workload. This means, of course, that the teacher donates all that work. This is a disadvantage because it will increase teacher resistance to teaching online courses. Worse, the teachers may simply not do the work and drop-out rates may then soar. Because the higher education environment in many schools now requires that teachers also be recruiters for their programs, student support in getting started in an online course becomes a big part of the success of the program—particularly for the continuing education program, but also for the distance degree programs.

The job is not done once the student is enrolled! The student is most likely to be lost during the first week of class and that is when the teacher needs to be most available to phone and e-mail students to provide any extra help they need getting into the course and getting started with their course work. Then, throughout the course, the teacher should be vigilant about continued participation of students. If a particular student's partici- pation begins to lag, the teacher needs to first e-mail and then phone that student to encourage continued participation in the course. With this approach, we have achieved a completion rate of approximately 90% over the past 5 years in our online continuing education program. Without this vigilance, we would have lost a significant number of these students along the way; I am quite sure we would have attrition rates in the usual range of 30% to 40% rather than in the 10% range. Unfortunately, this requires extra work from the teacher and to my knowledge no schools award extra workload credit to higher education teachers for these efforts. Perhaps few faculty are actually doing this kind of student monitoring and support work; perhaps that is the reason so many schools are re- porting such high attrition rates.

Seventh, *issues of copyright, privacy, security, plagiarism, and au- thentication of student work constitute special problems for Internet courses.* On-campus courses have library reserve desks where a teacher can place a copy of a journal article, book, or other material that he or she wishes to share with students. Copyright laws forbid the teacher, bookstore, and copy center to make copies for all the students unless permission is obtained from the publisher of the material, and sometimes a royalty must be paid to the copyright owner. Of course, in the library, each student can make a personal copy, so the effect is the same as if the teacher or bookstore were making copies. In a Web-based course this approach does not work. The teacher or university must make contact with the owner of the copyright and either buy reprints or pay a royalty for uploading a copy for all the students to use or download or copy as they see fit. With reprints, the students buy the reprints with their course packet (that includes texts and other materials purchased through the bookstore).

Faculty always have to be concerned that students may submit purchased term papers and other students' work as their own. There are public sites on the Web that sell papers for this very purpose. This is a serious problem in America. One of the reasons our educational system is so well respected and that our students are marketable all over the world is the rigor of our coursework. If students begin to pass with high grades without doing the necessary work to earn the grade, a college degree from an American university will soon become less valuable. All parts of the system must guard against cheating and grade inflation. Employers hire graduates with the understanding that the college degree is backed by a considerable knowledge base and certain writing, critical thinking, and analytic skills. Unfortunately, Web courses do not offer any better protections against dishonesty than do classroom courses. In fact, for exams, the Web-based courses do have one disadvantage: closed-book exams are much more difficult to achieve. Also, it can be difficult to prevent several students from getting together and taking the exams together. In a traditional classroom, the teacher knows who the students are; in very large exam rooms, sometimes students must present their picture ID, which is checked against the class list.

There are some ways to help ensure an honest exam. In the past, we have had students identify a teacher, department chair, or other school official in a community college or university near the student's home to proctor the exam. The student had to contract with the proctor and provide us with the proctor's name, title, address, and phone number 30 days in advance of the exam. We verified the identity of the proctor by calling the school and checking on his or her credentials and then calling the proctor to discuss a mutually agreeable exam process. We then faxed the exam to the proctor the day prior to the exam, and the proctor faxed the completed exam back to the course instructor immediately after the exam was completed. There are companies such as the American College Testing Corporation (ACT) that will provide a computer and proctor for exams for a fee. Of course, these preparations are extra work, but these examples show that there are ways to accomplish proctored examinations for Web-based courses.

Another method that has worked well is the use of integrative essay exams. We develop exam questions that require the student to integrate and analyze course information. These are open-book, open-notes exams, and we allow several days for completion. Several of our students have commented that the exams took 6 to 8 hours to complete. However, they also said they learned a huge amount from the exams because the questions helped them think through the meaning of the content in the text and class notes.

Finally, *the teacher needs to be intimately involved with assisting first-time students to get started successfully and to work to keep students from dropping out of the classes.* This is especially true of continuing education courses, but is also true with degree-seeking students. In my courses, I check every day the first week the course is available. If a student hasn't signed in and put up his or her introduction by the third or fourth day, I'm concerned. I will e-mail that student via their home e-mail address or phone the student to find out if there is an access problem I can help with. Occasionally I discover the student was having a problem getting into the course, or couldn't make some aspect of the technology work, or perhaps was just confused about the start date. Had I not contacted the student, the problem might have led to the student's dropping out due to falling too far behind at the start of the semester. Only the teacher knows if the student is active in the course, so only the teacher can perform this student retention marketing activity. This is a fairly new role for most higher education faculty, and some don't feel it is a suitable role for them. Although it is understandable that faculty might resist taking on this kind of back-end marketing activity in an already full faculty workload, it is essential to the success of many online educational programs.

THREE COMMON MYTHS OF WEB-BASED COURSES

Myth 1: Faculty Can Accommodate More Students by Using Technology

This myth is particularly damaging to a school's efforts to get a program started. It frightens teachers because they actually need *small* classes to start with. A Web-based course may increase the size of those classes that tend to have a small local enrollment. The distance opportunity increased our Informatics course from 7 to 25 the year after we began offering it online. The point is that the Web format will help fill classes. It does *not* reduce faculty workload for a given course—it may in fact, increase the workload involved in teaching a course.

A Web-based course does *change* the distribution of the way work happens for a course. For a new course, most schools want all the course modules to be completely written and up on the Web the first day of class. Therefore, the front-end work is intense. In a typical classroom course, teachers design a course in advance, but they actually write the lectures week-by-week the first time they teach it. So the work is spread out over a semester. As the teacher writes lectures, meets with students, and returns phone calls, he or she is also writing the lectures each week. This is why a new course preparation is so much work, regardless of whether it is online or in a classroom. For the Web course, all that module development is done in advance. So during the semester, the workload in development is reduced. Subsequent times the course is taught, the Web course must be updated in advance of the course. Classroom courses can be updated weekly.

For all course modalities, however, students' questions and concerns must be addressed regularly and in a timely fashion, and papers must be graded as they come in. Where a Web course can become overwhelming is in the class discussion area. An on-campus course class discussion is very limited. It must fit into the classroom hours. This is not so with a Web-based course and this fact can create a real problem for the instructor.

In one of my Web courses with 26 students, I had more than 1,276 student entries on the discussion board in the first 3 months of the class. That can become a serious workload for the teacher—and for the students. In this aspect of Web courses, the workload for a Web course can greatly exceed the workload of an on-campus course. And it is this aspect of Web courses—and the need to give personal attention to students in Web courses—that makes class sizes of 60 to 100 or greater a poor idea for Web-based courses unless there are teaching assistants to assist the primary course instructor in keeping that personal touch. The number of items in the course discussion area will be so huge that nobody could possibly read them all, much less respond to those who ask the teacher a question.

Even in ordinary size classes of 20 to 30, the class discussion must be managed in a Web-based course. Here are some ways to limit the course discussion:

1. Ask students to send supportive comments to each other via private e-mail. Many times, students want to praise each other for a particularly good entry on the discussion board. Unfortunately, if 26 people enter the comment, "I really agree with your item!" a great deal of time is wasted on those comments. And everybody ends up *having* to read those supportive comments if they are put up as public items. So in my initial instructions to students, I ask them to send those kinds of comments to each other via private course e-mail. Web-CT (the course software we use) allows the students to either REPLY—put the reply on the public conference so everybody

in the class sees it; or to REPLY PRIVATELY—send the reply only to the writer of the item that so impressed the reader. I require students to send responses of interest only to the writer privately in order to save everybody else time. And I enforce that by gently (and privately) sending a reminder to anyone who publicly posts a personal-type response.

2. Break larger classes into work groups and give each work group a private discussion forum, and then have discussion assignments divided by work groups. That way you may have a bigger reading workload as teacher, but the students will not have so much to read. Each student reads only his or her own group's items in the private forums. Students do not even see other private forums in Web-CT, so their reading load is kept reasonable. In fact, if my class is large, I use private forums only for their private group work sessions. In that case, I tell them I will not be reading items in their private forums and I keep a few public forums for items for the whole class. Then I tell students that if they have things they want me to read, they must either e-mail me or post in a class-wide public forum. In the latter instance, final papers are either e-mailed to the instructor or posted in a separate place in the course.

3. I do want students to network with each other. But this means private, non–course-related conversations. Busy students may resent having their time wasted on such conversations when they are in a hurry, so I create a private networking forum for this purpose. Sometimes I name it "Coffee House" or "Networking Forum." But I warn students I will not usually read that forum, and ask them to keep non–course-related conversations in that forum. I encourage them to use it liberally to share ideas about their jobs, fun vacations, recipes, or anything else they want to use it for. But nobody has to read it, and everybody is welcome to use it for anything that isn't related to course work. That saves a great deal of wear and tear on nerves. Teachers need to be aware that even if they do not complain, some people get angry at having to read non–course-related conversations in the mandatory forums. The reality is, students will get involved in non–work-related conversations in the course. So rather than trying to eliminate those discussions, I just have a place for them to happen. So far, it has worked extremely well.

4. Now, what if you have the opposite problem? Nobody is discussing anything! That is a function of poor course design. You must design your course so that students *have* to begin having discussions the very first day of class. My first course assignment requires the students to enter their introduction on the Conference Center. What you ask them to enter is up to you, but I ask at the minimum: name, city and state location, home phone and home e-mail address

in case I or somebody in their private group needs to reach them urgently; their nursing specialty, what kind of unit they work in, and their job. Then they are free to introduce whatever else they wish others to know about them. Of course I put my own introduction in the Conference Center first. I tell them a bit about my educational background and job experiences (things I tell my on-campus students so they too know who their teacher is). Then, to make it a more personal experience, I add information about my husband and children, pets and favorite hobbies, and perhaps recent vacations. Depending on the kind and level of the course, I may share information about research projects, recent publications and other scholarly activities (especially if it is a PhD course).

After the introduction, there should be regular assignments for course topics they are to discuss on the Conference Center. A percentage of the grade should be allocated to the class discussions. Students who are actively engaged in the class discussion seldom drop out of the course.

This brings up the issue of how often the teacher needs to enter items on the Conference Center and to respond to items students place on the Conference Center. Although each teacher needs to find his or her own level of effective response, at a minimum the teacher should respond to *every* student's introduction with a personalized welcome response. Because you are not face-to-face, it is doubly important to make each student feel personally recognized and welcome to your class. I cannot imagine a course in which I failed to put at least three to four items or responses per week on the Conference Center, just so students know that I'm present and active with them in the course. Typically, I will use the Conference Center to share ideas and information that is not in the text or available in online readings.

Students want and need the benefit of your experience and special knowledge. They cannot be expected to use the class discussion area if you are not active in the class in that area. I tend to teach by telling stories from my own nursing experience. In my course evaluations, students have said they really appreciate those stories because they learn so much from hearing about real situations that I have lived through. And the stories can be ones you have heard from colleagues or have read in professional journals. But in some way, share of yourself, your knowledge and experience. That is why they have a teacher.

Myth 2: Using Technology Saves the Institution Money

Someday, this may not be a fiction. Someday, the cost of classroom space and utilities and maintenance and other physical space costs will be reduced by online courses. Unfortunately, those cost savings today are generally not fully recognized. Too many administrators believe the cost savings will come from having huge class sizes because physical classroom limitations will not apply to online classes, and that money can be saved if one teacher can handle a much larger number of students. However, for some of the reasons listed above, programs that are successful will not generally have extremely large student-to-faculty ratios. If the students cannot get timely responses to their questions, they will find another school that provides sufficient faculty time. Some schools hope to make money by attracting more out-of-state students, who pay much higher tuition. Only time will prove this true or false. Today, many schools offer in-state tuition or reduced out-of-state tuition to Internet students in order to fill classes. Over time, we suspect that a few prestigious schools offering full degree programs will be able to fill Internet classes, even at out-of-state tuition costs. Schools that offer only isolated courses or whose reputation is not world-class will have to offer cheaper tuition to fill classes. Money also can be saved if the number of buildings (and attendant maintenance costs) can be reduced. This is where the real cost savings are most likely to be realized. Internet students do not use the classrooms or student activity buildings that traditional campuses must provide. We suspect that eventually, if enough students opt for online courses, the number and size of buildings can be reduced (or more likely, given the need for lifelong continuing education, not expanded).

The myth that technology saves the faculty members' time is not as prominent as it was in the late 1990s. The development time needed for a Web-based course is now recognized as much greater than that for a traditional course. Faculty workload must be greatly reduced when a teacher is first learning to teach online. The first time I taught a course online, I spent approximately 30 hours per week on that one course for a whole semester. I was learning to use the technology, honing my HTML skills (this was in 1995 before Front Page or other Web authoring programs were available and certainly before Web-CT or Blackboard was available), developing and trying out new ways to offer material, and experiencing the inefficiency of any beginner. Today, that same course can be taught much more efficiently. As an experienced online teacher, I spend about the same amount of time preparing for and teaching an online course as I do for on-campus courses. Of course, because I can teach the online course at my convenience rather than on the university's class schedule, it sometimes seems easier to teach that course than to teach on-campus courses.

Myth 3: Online Teachers Cannot Know Students Personally

Many teachers think if they cannot see the students, they cannot get to know them. *Au contraire!* I get to know many of my Internet students much better than I know many of my on-campus students. Online teachers may or may not have the benefit of video technology, or even have a photograph of the student, but they certainly can communicate personally with each student at least once per week. Human personalities come across in computer communications quite nicely. There is a feeling of equality about the Web that many students don't experience in person. Web students can be given permission to address us by our first names; they often share their personal lives with us. I continue to hear from both online and on-campus students today, even though they completed course work years ago. That long-term relationship does not always happen, but it adds greatly to the joy of teaching as a career choice. Teachers develop as great a fondness for Internet students as for on-campus students. (The only thing you cannot do is hug your Internet students.) Otherwise, the teaching-learning experience can be equally intense.

KEY ISSUES IN DELIVERING CONTENT TO DISTANCE STUDENTS

Some key issues involved in using the Internet to deliver distance courses include (a) knowing your customer, (b) development of a student facilitation model of teaching, (c) preservation of academic standards, and (d) registration and enrollment issues. There is much to think through in each of these areas if a high-quality, credible educational program is to be offered through the Internet.

Who Is the Customer?

In this medium, more than in any other, students are your customers. Clearly, each student must be given a good education and should receive good service from the entire educational institution, from the registrar and teacher to the support staff. As more colleges and universities get into the business of offering online courses, students have more choices. Thus, it is important to market to potential students, and part of marketing is excellent service. The student should be able to discover your online program through trade journals, Internet search engines, and professional contacts. Every university should have an online registration and enrollment system. Students should not have to use the U.S. postal service (called "snail mail" by e-mail users). One of the problems for graduate students is the need to contact their undergraduate universities by mail to get transcripts. It is important that universities develop a system whereby a student can pay for a transcript online with a credit card, and the university simply e-mails the transcript to the graduate school or department where the student plans to enroll. In our experience, this transcript issue has caused too many delays in enrollment.

Students are your most immediate customers. They are neither your only nor your most important customer. The most important customer is the future employer of your graduates. It is important for *all* faculty to maintain a relationship with community employers, and if possible, with the national employer community. We regularly meet with local directors of nursing and agency CEOs to talk about what they think we should include in our courses. We have department meetings with these people to consult with them on the full curriculum. Maintaining close contact with the world in which your students are expected to function is essential to the quality of your content.

Ultimately, your customer is all of society. In publicly owned schools, taxes provide at least some of the support for overhead, faculty salaries, and other costs. Even if none of the costs are tax-supported, the value of your educational offerings will ultimately be judged by society's respect for your graduates. It is important to maintain the goodwill of the public because schools are social institutions. If your graduates have poor skills, ultimately your university's reputation will suffer; and parents, teachers, high-school counselors, and other advisors will not encourage students to seek their education from your school. Both faculty and students are ultimately public relations representatives for your school. It is everybody's job to ensure that a degree from your institution is treated with respect and admiration everywhere.

Maintain Extremely High Academic Standards

Students must leave your course with marketable new knowledge and skills. If the degree your university confers is not backed by solid knowledge and skills, the value of a degree from your institution will decline. We once knew of a vice president of nursing who would not hire nursing graduates with master's degrees from the local university. She claimed that their degrees were given too easily and that the students could not communicate well in writing. She further noted that if their skills were not a significant improvement over the skills of the nurses with a basic nursing education, she could not justify paying them more. In another case, where there was much cheating in a computer programming department, the university began having trouble placing students in local businesses. Students found they had to leave town to find a job because local employers had no faith in their work skills and work habits.

The moral of these two stories is that although there may be pressure from a few students to give good grades for poor performance, giving in to that pressure is ultimately an unsuccessful strategy. Unfortunately, those few students can create havoc in a teacher's life. Even more unfortunately, some administrators too quickly assume that the teacher is at fault if a student complains about a teacher to the school's administration. The vast majority of students are motivated to work hard and they value the new skills they learn in well-designed, academically rigorous courses. In fact, good students will rightly complain if a course doesn't teach them anything new. It is essential that administrators listen carefully to student complaints and discriminate between complaints that have validity and complaints that are based on a student wanting an unfairly high grade.

There should be a peer review process in place so that the quality of courses can be checked. Obviously, student evaluations of a course are one important source of information about the quality of a course (either online or on-campus). But they should not be the only source of information about course quality. Other expert instructors should review every online course, ideally before it goes live, to ensure that its quality and content are excellent, that it flows smoothly, and that there is the right amount of work for credit hours awarded.

University Faculty Evaluation Committees

Such groups must be extremely careful when interpreting student evaluations of faculty and courses. In our opinion, the student's evaluation should be linked with the student's course grade. If it can be demonstrated that evaluations correlate highly with student grades, then only the A students' course evaluations should be considered in faculty evaluations. Faculty members are smart, and if they find that their job evaluations and merit raises are dependent on making every student happy with them, grade inflation is the only possible result. Ultimately, grade inflation is the fault of the system, not of the individual teacher. This is true of all courses, but especially of online courses because of the great personal discipline required of distance students.

Techniques to Make Learning Easier

Make difficult content easier to learn by reducing the red tape and unnecessary bureaucracy as much as possible, not by "dumbing down" your content and expectations. Be meticulous about organizing the material in such a way that learning proceeds logically. Avoid jumping back and forth among topics. Make the course and module objectives explicit, clear, and measurable. For example, avoid objectives such as "The student will understand how to start an IV." A better objective might be "The student will list the five principles of starting an IV and will successfully demonstrate the technique." Then break down the module into sub-objectives that incorporate the five principles. Course and module objectives must be behavioral, measurable, and clearly linked to both individual class session objectives and to assignments, projects, and examinations.

Difficult content should be broken up into small bites. To the extent possible, liberally sprinkle it with visuals. Most people are highly visual learners; photos, graphics, and, if possible, videos should be incorporated into their learning materials (Horton, 2000). Difficult content is almost always somewhat boring to read, so the teacher can add interest if visuals are colorful. Color attracts the eye and holds the interest. Whenever possible, create small learning activities that will help the student learn difficult content in small steps. For example, the nursing process is a fairly difficult one, so it is taught in separate steps. First, students spend a lot of time learning different assessment techniques. Then they learn various nursing diagnoses and nursing interventions together. The interventions and assessment techniques are fun to learn, but making nursing diagnoses—a complex, critical thinking, cognitive process—is more difficult and not nearly as much fun to learn. So it is taught throughout while the more enjoyable techniques are taught intermittently. In this way, students are able to put it all together so that they can provide comprehensive care to patients.

Consider this piecemeal approach to teaching difficult content. Break long modules into shorter units. Associate fun learning activities with each unit and give the students sufficient time to complete each unit, but insist that they make steady progress on unit completion. I try not to be too lenient about late assignments unless the student has a bona fide excuse like a serious illness or a death in the family. "I fell behind" isn't acceptable. It isn't helpful to students to let them fall behind and many students need the discipline of knowing there is a penalty for late assignments.

Design Screens With Eye Appeal

Colors should provide good contrast so that the student can read text. Never use pastel text on a light background. Use large print and easy-to-read print fonts, such as Arial or Times Roman, so that students don't get eyestrain. Color, font style and size, and movement (such as that found in animation) can be used to draw attention to important points and maintain interest. Present content in the same order you listed the objectives to make it easy for students to follow the learning trajectory you planned for your course. Incorporate graphics, videos, photos, and other visuals as much as possible (so long as they enhance learning) because people respond to visual learning aids. Never make the screen busy with "cutesy" things like butterflies in the background or other things that distract from your content.

Make Learning Fun

Develop or search out public-domain case studies that make learning difficult content fun. A teacher should strive to be an entertainer as well as a conveyer of knowledge. Remember the history of the television show *All in the Family*. It used comedy, lovable and sometimes unlovable characters, and drama to make some very important points about human dignity and justice. Even people who were reared in racist environments watched that show despite the fact that its content was diametrically opposed to their personal beliefs. It probably brought home the unfairness and wrongness of racial and ethnic discrimination to many people who would otherwise never have questioned their beliefs.

People learn and retain knowledge better when it is fun to learn. We have had games in our Informatics courses in which the students had a contest to find the best sites for things like ergonomics research. In order to make learning to use the online library more fun, we have a treasure hunt in which the teacher provides hints about a particular journal article, and the students use the hints to do an online OVID search to try and find a nursing article that fits all the hints. In order to find the article, they have to learn to limit their search by years, topics, and full-text papers. We also had a game in which students were asked to find one credible and one untrustworthy site for a particular medical problem. They had to search out the Internet and the professional literature to find out who the author was, if the author had a professional affiliation with a credible institution, and if he or she was providing professional information or personal opinion. Several students have told us that after playing the game, they never again assumed the validity of something on the Web; they always check out the source. Some things will always require hard study and work. (Children still have to memorize the multiplication tables.) But teachers should always remember that learning is much easier and better retained when teachers and parents can make a game of learning.

Design Course to Achieve Stated Objectives

Ensure that class "lectures," case studies, and assignments are designed to assist the student to achieve the stated objectives. Students legitimately dislike busywork. They resent assignments if they cannot understand why they are doing them. Good teachers give assignments that are designed to meet explicit learning objectives, and the learning materials should make clear what each part of the course contributes to the students' learning process.

Real-Time Requirements

Decide whether to require any real-time learning experiences. Chat rooms and audio-conferencing technology can be effective ways to provide for class discussion and can give teachers important outlets for their need to personally share their expertise with students in a direct way. However, real-time experiences may be inconvenient in the extreme for students who live in widely different time zones. If the student body is limited to North and South America, a reasonable time for a real-time experience might be noon Central Standard Time (CST). That would have students in the east online at 1:00 p.m. Students on Mountain Standard Time would get online at 11:00 a.m.; while students on Pacific Standard Time would join the class at 10:00 a.m., Alaska at 9:00 a.m., the Aleutian Islands at 8:00 a.m. Students in Hawaii would have to sign on at 7:00 a.m. A real-time experience scheduled for 8:00 a.m. Eastern Standard Time requires Californians to sign on at 5:00 a.m. and Hawaiians at 2:00 a.m. Clearly, a course that has students from around the world must carefully consider any real-time experiences.

Develop Assignments and Explicit Grading Criteria

Make assignments and grading criteria available to students in the syllabus. An advantage of Internet courses is that they can allow students to plan their class work schedules at their own convenience. Distance students often are people with erratic and demanding work schedules who work in nontraditional ways. For example, a student may have no time to work on the course 1 week but may spend 2 or 3 entire days another week. Instructors also must control their schedules. Therefore, a student submitting an assignment early does not necessarily mean the faculty has to grade it early. Students like quick feedback, so the syllabus should clearly state that early papers may not be graded until the due date because due dates are one way teachers plan their own work schedules.

By all means, have due dates. Due dates help students discipline themselves to get projects done. The teacher should consider having grade penalties for late work. However, working adults will sometimes need 2- or 3-day extensions. We find it most helpful to require students to ask for extensions and always include a new due date for the extension. Procrastinators may be poorly disciplined, but they also may be people who have great need for flexibility because of work and family demands. The most successful attitude is directed toward facilitating students' work, not toward punitive actions. We contract, cajole, and encourage students to get their work in. We are not comfortable threatening students with an F grade except in the most extreme cases. For example, we must remind students of the consequence of noncompletion when they still haven't completed their work more than a month or two after the end of the course. Some students do find after they enroll that they simply do not have what it takes to complete an online course. Despite our flexibility, it is always students' responsibility to manage their time.

Withdrawal dates should be generous. People should have at least until midterm to withdraw without receiving an F. The teacher should schedule enough assignments during the first half of the course so that a substantial workload hits in the first 4 weeks. That way, students will have a chance to determine early if they cannot handle the workload. If they aren't going to be able to do their work, and the course is group-work–dependent, the student can withdraw and the teacher can make adjustments to work assignments. To repeat, it is best for the teacher to view the relationship as facilitative, not punitive.

Take an Active Role in Facilitating Class Discussion

Most students will not use the discussion facilities unless it is a class requirement. They begin by greatly preferring to communicate only with the instructor via e-mail. This practice *must* be discouraged. Students need to use each other as resources, and teachers must protect their own time. It is not efficient to answer the same question 25 times to individuals. We always copy student content questions onto the discussion board and respond to them there. Soon, students learn to use the board for content questions.

The best technique we have found is to have a discussion-board assignment the very first week. This approach also helps Internet support personnel manage their time. We simply let them know that the first week or two students will be required to use the discussion board, so that is when most of those technical questions will arise. Some students will have to be nudged occasionally with an e-mail suggesting that they make some entries on the board. In most classes, there will be some eager users and some who just do not care to participate much in the class discussion. However, we have had people who were very quiet in an on-campus course become the busiest users of the discussion board. Shyness is not the barrier here. Students' time pressures may be a factor.

HINTS FOR GOOD WEB-COURSE DESIGN

- Do not get too fancy. A good design is a simple one. Limit the use of frames technology unless it is central to the navigation scheme.

- Legibility is extremely important. The user should not have to squint to read your text. Large, familiar, readable serif fonts (such as Times Roman) or sans serif fonts (such as Arial) work best.

- Provide users with a guide to where they are in relation to the entire page. This can be accomplished with visual indicators, page numbers, and a variety of other techniques.

- Be consistent. Provide users with the same navigation features in predictable locations on the screen. Do not get fancy or move things around. Decide on a template and stick with it.

- Provide basic information about the course and instructor. For instance, an instructor bio with information on how to contact the instructor by e-mail and phone is critical. Use the school or company logo on the opening page. Identify the course and provide an area for visitors to e-mail for further information.

- Create an index page that provides users with an easy way to get to specific information.

- Provide users with links to support services, embedded into your course; for instance, links to the library, bookstore, registrar's office, financial aid, and the like.

- Avoid embedding fancy things like Java-based applets (calculators, etc.) unless you are sure the students have a browser that is Java-enabled.

- Make the course multisensory, multidimensional. Do not limit the course to being a "computer textbook" but instead consider using the power of the Internet to enhance the course with audio, video, photos, animation, interactive testing, and so on.

- Develop an evaluation/feedback instrument for the course. Encourage feedback following every unit or module.

- The course home page is a marketing tool. Obtain professional consultation and design services to be sure it is very attractive and interesting. Of course, it must be easy to find.

MARKET YOUR COURSE

- Faculty responsible for the course should ensure that an attractive, informative course home page is created and maintained as a marketing tool.

- Register the course with as many search engines as possible.

- Register the course with *The World Lecture Hall*.

- Be sure that program fliers and other promotional materials include the course home-page address as well as a course listing and course description, and a phone number for the customer to call.

- Try to get a paper or news article about your course published in local, regional, and national professional newspapers or journals.

- Advertise your Web-based educational offerings in magazines and journals targeted at your potential student audience.

- Be sure that your university, college, and department home pages have prominent links to your course.

- Be sure that your course home page has links to the school's admissions and enrollment Web pages.

- Your home page should have a clearly marked link to online course registration (if it exists) or to an e-mail address where potential students can request enrollment forms.

MARKETING THROUGHOUT THE COURSE

- Make sure you provide the personal touch to your students throughout the teaching of the course.

- Communicate regularly on the conference center.

- Be liberal with personal e-mails to your students.

- If any student's participation begins to lag, communicate personally to let them know you care about them and do not want to lose them. Find out what is wrong and what *you* need to do or can do to make it possible for that student to continue in the course.

- Be supportive. These are adults and very difficult life situations sometimes happen to them. Parents get sick or die, they themselves (perhaps being older) may get sick or need surgery, or some may lose their jobs during a course—any number of disasters can happen. It is almost never useful for them to drop out of the course. So extend deadlines or do whatever you can to help them complete the course and earn the academic credit they have paid for.

- Be kind. These are adult learners. They need a coach, facilitator, guide, and friend along their learning path.

- The purpose of assignment due dates is twofold. First, they are there to help the students self-regulate and get work done in a timely, step-by-step fashion. Second, they are there to help you give regular feedback to students. Neither of those purposes is consistent with a stern or punitive "parental" stance. So if a student has a problem with a due date, be liberal with extensions. But to be consistent with the purpose, be sure to have them set new, reasonable due dates and stick with them.

NOTES

1. A rule of thumb for graduate school is as follows: For every credit hour, allow 3 hours of work outside class for homework, reading, library time, and student projects. Therefore, a 3-credit course should take the student 12 hours per week—3 hours of class time and 9 hours outside class. The rule for undergraduate courses is generally 2 hours of work for every credit hour plus in-class time. These are only general rules; students who have difficulty with the material may need more time, and students with a special aptitude or prior training may need less time.

REFERENCES

Heinke, H., & Russum, J. (2001). Factors influencing attrition in a corporate distance education program. *Education at a Distance Journal, 14*(11). Retrieved May 24, 2005 from http://www.chartula.com/attrition.pdf

Horton, W. (2000). *Designing Web-based training.* New York: Wiley.

Parker, A. (1999). A study of variables that predict dropout from distance education. *International Journal of Educational Technology, 1*(2), 20–23.

Phipps, R., & Merisotis, J. (1999). *What's the difference? A review of contemporary research on the effectiveness of distance learning in higher education.* Washington, DC: Council for Higher Education Accreditation.

Russell, T. (1998). *No Significant Difference: Phenomenon as Reported in 248 Research Reports, Summaries and Papers* (4th ed.). Raleigh: North Carolina State University.

Sparrow, C. (2004). Education and learning to learn. *The Challenge Forum.* Retrieved May 24, 2005 from http://www.chforum.org/library/xc143.html

Thompson, E. (1997, February). Distance education drop-out: What can we do? In R. Popisil & L. Willcoxson (Eds.), *Learning through teaching: Proceedings of the 6th Annual Teaching Forum* (pp. 324–332). Perth, Australia: Murdoch University. Retrieved May 24, 2005 from http://lsn.curtin.edu.au/tlf/tlf1997/contents.html

Zolkos, R. (1999, October). Online education getting good grades: Despite high attrition, online courses seen as possible alternative to the classroom. *Business Insurance,* p. 40-A.

CHAPTER 3

Supporting Learner Success

Carla L. Mueller and Diane M. Billings

As nurses and nursing students increasingly seek access to academic and continuing education and require convenient times and places for educational pursuits, learning at a distance is becoming the norm rather than the exception. Being a member of a distance education (DE) learning community requires changes in approaches to learning on the part of the student and additional services for technical, academic, personal, and career support on the part of the institution providing the educational offering. Unfortunately, support for the distance learner has not been widely studied (Oehlkers & Gibson, 2001). The purposes of this chapter are to identify the needs for learner support in DE courses and programs and to discuss strategies for providing the resources to support learner success.

LEARNER SUPPORT

Learner support in DE "includes the many forms of assistance that are designed to remove barriers (situational, institutional, dispositional, and informational) and promote academic success. Examples of such services are preadmission counseling, academic advising, financial aid, learning skills instruction, child care and much more" (Potter, 1998, p. 60). Pre-enrollment support includes information about programs and courses involved, assessment of whether DE is the appropriate learning modality for the students' circumstances and learning style, assessment of computer skills, assessment of prior learning, academic advising, and orientation to the particulars of the distance learning delivery method.

Once enrolled in DE, students face many changes that can have short- and long-term effects on their lives. Schlossberg (1984) reports that adult behavior is determined by transition, not by age. Schlossberg's transition theory facilitates understanding of adult students in transition by providing insight into factors related to the transition to a new way of learning and use of technology. It can provide information regarding the degree of impact that the transition will have and the assistance that students will need to cope with the transition. Schlossberg noted that four areas influence students' ability to cope with transition related to higher education: situation, self, support, and strategies. Academic institutions can influence the *situation* by helping students to view the role changes initiated by college enrollment in DE courses as positive and helping students to manage stress. Faculty can influence *self* by facilitating students' access to psychological resources. This is critical because many student problems are not course related, but are personal problems (Robinson, 1981). Institutional support, computer training, and opportunities for students to develop a support group via their DE courses can positively influence *support* for students during their transition to DE. To influence *strategies* positively, colleges and universities must have effective learning resources available to meet the needs of students taking DE courses for the first time. Phillips and Kelly (2001) believe "adult learner services compliment the teaching process and should be an integral component of a distance education program." Although support is often a set of standardized services, Granger (1989) and Oehlkers and Gibson (2001) encourage identifying individual learner needs and providing a program that meets the needs of the students.

Successful transition to DE, therefore, depends on learners being oriented to the unique aspects of teaching and learning at a distance and to the multiple avenues for support. This includes informing the learner about the DE course; orienting the learner to the technology, use of learning resources, the DE learning community, and the role of the learner; providing technical support; and assisting the student to develop personal and study support systems.

Recently the development of learner support in DE has paralleled and reflected the change in conceptualization of education as transmission of pre-packaged knowledge to that of a dynamic transformative process, focusing on developmental constructivist models of teaching and learning and finding ways to engage the learner as an active and central participant in the learning process (Brindley, von Ossietzky, & Paul, 2004, p. 2).

INFORMING THE LEARNER ABOUT COURSES

Because DE courses represent a significant departure from on-campus courses, students must be informed that the course will use DE technology prior to registration (Harasim, Hiltz, Teles, & Turoff, 1996). Providing information prior to the course gives students an opportunity to determine if this course will be appropriate for their learning needs, to determine what resources they will need to acquire or access (e.g., purchasing a computer or locating the videoconference outreach site), and to prepare themselves for new ways of learning.

DE may not be an appropriate option for every student, and providing students an opportunity to assess their own needs and learning styles may alert them to their own ability to be successful. Additionally, DE courses involve active learning, participation, and assignments that involve writing. Potential students may find it helpful to be informed of the demands of the DE course and the changes in student roles before they enroll (Billings & Bachmeier, 1994). The Distance Learning Technologies Group has developed a self-evaluation for potential online students that can help students decide if a Web-based program is for them. Questions include the following: "Do you feel that high quality learning can take place without going to a traditional educational facility? Are you a self-motivated and self-disciplined person? Are you comfortable communicating in writing?" (Bedore, Bedore, & Bedore, 1998, p. 17). A questionnaire entitled "Is Distance Learning a Good Match for You?" is available online at http://www.pbs.org/campus/003_Advice/003-06.html and may help students assess how well DE courses fit their needs.

Several strategies can be used to inform the learner about the DE course, such as including the information in the university bulletin of courses, providing information on the school of nursing Web site, and mailing or e-mailing information letters. Some schools use a learner assessment, posted on the school Web site, which prospective students can use to determine if they have the technical skills (particularly computer literacy and Internet research skills), writing skills, educational background, readiness for the self-directed learning and independence needed for success in DE courses, family and employer support, and the time required for the course.

At the beginning of any new DE program, it is helpful to use more than one strategy to keep the student informed about the DE options. For example, Cobb and Mueller (1998) found that although students had been informed about computer literacy requirements in the course bulletin, a follow-up letter was helpful in giving them further information and giving times of classes that students could take to increase their skill level.

ORIENTING LEARNERS TO DISTANCE EDUCATION

A comprehensive orientation program is critical to the success of any DE program. The type of orientation will depend on the learner, the course content, and the DE delivery system used, but in general it should include orientation to the technology, how to access and use the learning resources required in the curriculum, the norms of the learning community, and strategies for successful learning.

Orientation to the Technology

The use of DE technology, particularly videoconferencing and Internet, requires special orientation to the technology tools, course management hardware and software, and other specific skills, such as using a video camera, sending e-mail attachments, copying to the clipboard, or using the course management hardware and software. Learners quickly must become self-sufficient, as technical support at the user site may or may not be readily accessible. For videoconference DE courses, this may involve learning how to establish the network connections and how to use the cameras at the reception site; for online courses this includes learning the use of the computer, browser, Internet service provider, and the course management software.

There are several approaches to orienting students to DE technology, and the selection of the approach should be based on the needs of the learners. One effective way to orient learners is in a hands-on immersion course of 4 to 6 hours (Harasim et al., 1996). This can be accomplished by having an orientation day on campus or at designated outreach sites. Others use videoconference technology or Internet chats to have all students together for the orientation. However, with learners geographically dispersed, it may not be feasible to have students come to a central location, and other strategies can be used.

Printed information that requires the least technological sophistication to send and use may be most appealing for some learners. The use of technology can be explained in user guides or handbooks illustrated with diagrams of equipment or sample computer screen views. User guides can be posted on the Web site. It is also helpful to have a practice course set up where students can test the hardware and software before the course begins.

Other strategies for orienting students to DE course-specific technology include using a videotape, CD-ROMs, online presentation systems, or streaming video or audio (or both) that demonstrates the use of the technology and provides orientation information. These strategies are more expensive to develop and deploy but may be helpful to students who cannot come to the campus.

Once students are oriented to the use of the DE technology, it may take as long as two to four class sessions for students to achieve sufficient skill proficiency to shift their primary focus to the content of the course. Faculty must be aware of the time it is taking students to be comfortable with the technology and should structure course activities that encourage both the development of technology skills and the acquisition and application of course concepts.

Orientation to the Norms for Participating in a DE Learning Community

As in any classroom, faculty and students establish the norms for appropriate behavior that facilitate participation and collegiality in the learning community. Norms should be established at the beginning of the class and reviewed and monitored as the course progresses. Norms include establishing and maintaining a sense of community, encouraging relevant participation, and respecting privacy, confidentiality, and the ethics of the learning community. Faculty can serve as a guide to membership in the community by modeling these behaviors (Bonk & Cunningham, 1998).

Establishing a sense of community in DE courses is necessary to overcome the barriers of distance and technology and, in some instances, lack of visual cues (audio conferencing, some Internet courses, and one-way-video TV-based courses). Community is established by introduction of all class members and if possible posting student pictures. Other group process strategies, such as creating a safe and supportive environment, encouraging participation from all students, and acknowledging responses, can be used to maintain the community (Harasim et al., 1996; Porter, 1997).

In Internet courses it is also important to establish norms for network etiquette (netiquette). Basic netiquette includes using student names, respecting differing views, being judicious in using humor, and avoiding insulting or hostile remarks (Harasim et al., 1996). There are several Internet netiquette sites that explain norms for class behavior; students can be referred there.

Participation is critical to active learning for individual students and the overall success of the course, and students should be oriented to the nuances of using DE technology to enable class participation as well as to the expectations for scholarly participation within the course. For example, in videoconference courses, students learn how to indicate that they wish to make a comment by dialing in to the discussion or releasing the "mute" function; in audio-based courses, students must learn how to listen for appropriate pauses in conversation in order to gain the "floor" (Henry, 1993). Participation in Internet courses is heavily text-based, often using threaded discussions, which can result in large numbers of messages, and students should be oriented to posting relevant comments and threading them appropriately.

Because learning outcomes depend on course participation and collaboration, expectations for participation should be made explicit at the beginning of the course. These expectations may include minimum numbers of contributions to course discussions or specifications for role activities when working in teams. Harasim et al. (1996) recommend motivating participation by making it a significant component of the course grade.

DE courses are more public than most classrooms, and norms for privacy, confidentiality, and ethical behavior are extremely important to the success of the learning community. Both faculty and students are responsible for affirming how these principles will be used in their course. For example, students and faculty should agree to confine discussion of privileged information to the course. It is also important to protect the privacy of clients and case studies that are discussed as examples of teaching points within the class; names and other identifying information should be withheld. Finally, school policies and ethical guidelines about the use of published material and respect for copyright and plagiarism should be observed.

Orientation to the Role of Learner in a Distance Education Course

The role of the learner is changing as the information technology tools of DE encourage active construction of knowledge, inquiry, critical thinking, reflection, collaboration, and use of learning resources and knowledge work tools. Students who are successful in DE courses are self-directed; independent; able to network with classmates, colleagues, and faculty;

and are well on their way to developing the skills of lifelong learning (Harasim et al., 1996). Faculty can assist students to develop these skills by guiding them to identify their learning needs and consider how those needs will be met, by negotiating roles, and by aligning support from families, employers, mentors, and experts.

Although the use of DE technology may make courses accessible and convenient, it also transforms learning into active and collaborative experiences that may be even more time-consuming than that experienced in some on-campus courses. Course management strategies are necessary to assure productive use of time. Faculty can assist students in planning for adequate time for the course by specifying learning outcomes and the amount of time needed to attain them. Students should be able to allocate sufficient time for course activities, identify study space, and learn to use the technology before class starts.

In learning communities, students assume responsibility for their own learning as well as for the success of the group. Students may have to be oriented to teams and collaborative work groups; faculty should mentor students in the formation of productive work groups and monitor the development of group process.

It is also important for students to understand their own learning styles and how they might be affected when taking a DE course. There are several learning styles inventories available, and some are now available on the Internet. Students can use them to assess their own learning style preferences and assume responsibility for adapting them to the DE learning environment.

Students with Special Needs

One of the emerging issues for DE programs is the accommodation of students with varying forms of disabilities. There has been little organized effort nationally in the United States to develop DE materials that are easily accessible to students with special needs. The U.S. government has only recently mandated that government Web sites must be accessible to those who are blind and mobility impaired (Farrell, 2001). General Web site design principles can be applied when designing DE materials for online posting and test sites are available to evaluate usability of Web-based materials that are developed (http://www.cast.org/bobby). Farrell (2001) reports that "disability interest groups such as the Blind Citizens Australia (http://wwww.bca.org.au) have made progress in producing appropriate principles for access to online courses. Links to information about adaptive computer products and publications can be found at http://www.makoa.org/computers.htm and can serve as a starting point for opening access to DE courses for students with special needs.

PROVIDING TECHNICAL SUPPORT

Although basic information about the technology can be provided during an orientation session, ongoing technical support is critical to supporting the learners and establishing successful learning communities. Technical help is particularly important during the first few weeks of the course, when specific problems with setting up technology and accessing the course are likely. Technical support is critical to student satisfaction with teaching effectiveness. Students perceive failure of the technology as failure of the instructor (Anderson, Banks, & Leary, 2002). Ideally, there should be a central technical support center that is available 24 hours a day, 7 days a week, to fulfill the DE promise of learning that is accessible *anytime, anywhere,* and *anyplace.* However, this increase in support comes at a steep institutional cost. "Macquarie University in Australia and the London School of Economics have partnered to provide 20 hour Help Desk support, without adding to institutional cost by utilizing the difference in time zones between the two institutions to provide coverage to each other's students" (Farrell, 2001).

The support center must be able to assist students with common software and hardware problems and to troubleshoot and establish connections to the course during peak hours. Many technical support centers have a toll-free number, a pager system, or e-mail that students can easily access. Course faculty must be certain students know how to contact the support center.

Technical support personnel are particularly critical for Internet courses and must be able to troubleshoot problems with hardware, software, Internet service providers, and network connections. When troubleshooting, the technical support team should ask students calling for assistance what type of computer equipment they are using. Cobb and Mueller (1998) found that despite instructions regarding the type of computer equipment necessary for Web-based courses, some students chose to continue using their home computer regardless of whether or not it met the hardware requirements for enrolling in the course, and these incompatibilities caused problems for course access.

Cartwright and Menkens (2002) found that many incoming students either overestimated their computer literacy skills or underestimated program technology requirements. Providing a variety of computer-skill–related information can ease students' transition into DE. Printed troubleshooting tips, online FAQ (frequently asked question) pages, and online flash movies demonstrating commonly used computer skills (e.g., e-mail attachments, using the "drop box" in a learning management system to turn in assignments, and Web searching) can decrease calls to the help desk for support, and increase students' satisfaction and comfort with the online learning environment. Cartwright and Menkens (2002) found that students also develop informal support networks of peers who are willing to assist other students with technical problems and questions. These peer networks work well and provide support just when students need it, as research supports that technical skills are often best learned in a subject-specific context, and hence integrated into the subject material of courses (Rossiter & Watters, 2000).

COURSE RESOURCE SUPPORT

Additional course resource support is needed for DE students. When students are far from campus, arrangements should be made with support offices to deal with DE students by some means other than face-to-face, or a special office should be set up to handle DE students. Providing a single contact point with in an area or a special office for DE students allows students to move directly to their questions and avoid explaining their situation each time. Kazmer (2002) found that DE students were more comfortable with the latter option because they knew the name of the person to call for assistance.

A review of activity logs for students in a program using a combination of videoconferencing and Web-based technology found that more than 40% of students were online between 10:00 p.m. and midnight during the week and during the weekend (Cartwright & Menkens, 2002). Therefore, support offices need to have hours outside the normal 8:30 a.m. to 5:00 p.m. to best meet the needs of DE students. Support staff are the silent heroes of DE and ensure that the myriad details required for program success are dealt with effectively.

There also should be provision for phone or online registration (including drop/add) and advising. Oehlkers and Gibson (2001) report that advisors are the "go-to person" when students have questions. Early assignment of an advisor and advising continuity enhances communication and problem solving.

E-mail Accounts

E-mail accounts should be set up for students prior to the beginning of the semester. The university must determine if students will be required to utilize the university e-mail system or can utilize their personal e-mail account through their Internet service provider. If the university system is required, it must be determined how access to the system can be facilitated in a cost-effective manner for students who live outside the university's local calling number. Faculty can obtain student e-mail addresses and set up a distribution list to facilitate communication to the class. Some Web-based courseware has a separate e-mail system set up within the courseware to allow students to have a separate e-mail account related to the Web course. This facilitates separation of e-mail and helps students who receive a large volume of e-mail on other accounts to find course-related messages in a timely manner.

Access and Use of Learning Resources

The use of learning resources changes in DE courses as students do not have easy access to the on-campus resources of libraries, learning laboratories, and other learning supports. Information about these learning resources should be developed and distributed to DE students to make sure they are aware of the services that exist and of how to access them. Information about these resources could be placed on the Web and linked to a common site for DE students, or printed material about the services could be developed and distributed to DE students.

A wide variety of learning resources are available to DE students. Using computer-supported collaborative tools, students have access to experts, mentors, professional colleagues, peers, and a variety of faculty; and a host of virtual patients, simulations, case studies, and authentic learning experiences are easily at hand. Faculty can assist students by guiding them through this resource-rich environment as they locate, retrieve, sort, organize, synthesize, evaluate, and critique relevant resources.

When designing courses and learning activities, faculty must be aware of the limits of the resources and students' ability to access them. Creating options and alternative learning activities gives students flexibility in the choice of learning resources. Faculty and students also have to be aware of the time required to access resources and plan for adequate access time within the time frame of the assignment or learning activity.

If the purpose of the DE course or program is to provide access and convenience for learners who are at a distance from the campus, faculty must consider differences in time zones, limits of local resources, and the extent to which the campus learning resources can be available to learners at a distance. In courses that span geography and cultures, faculty must also be aware of when holidays and weekends occur and how time differences will influence access to resources. Faculty also should determine whether current office hours and modes of contact fit the needs of DE students and make adjustments as needed.

Library Access

A single point of access to library services would guide students to available resources. As student-centered learning communities evolve and as increasing information is available on the Internet, learning resources are even more abundant and convenient. For example, literature searches, databases such as MedLine and CINAHL, and full-text articles are all accessible through the Internet. Additionally, many nursing journals are now online, often available through the school of nursing or university library. Faculty also can place links to these resources within the course or on a resource page of the school of nursing Web site.

Library access continues to be critical to enable students to complete the research for assignments in DE courses. Convenience proved more influential in the selection of a library to use than the resources that were available. DE students reported that they usually needed library resources quickly, with nearly 80% needing material within 1 week (Butler, 1997). DE students may never be on campus or may be on campus in a limited fashion; thus, alternative ways of obtaining library access must be developed so that students can access resources in a timely manner. Students and faculty lack basic awareness about the library services available to DE students; thus, it is critical that information about the library's services be publicized. A survey by the University of Minnesota Libraries (Butler, 1997) found that although most students reported adequate computer access, "these students reported rarely to never using these technologies . . . for activities related to library research" (p. 3).

Technical help in using the library via the Internet is particularly important. The library should be able to assist students with common problems and facilitate their obtaining the references they need to complete their assignments. Many libraries utilize a toll-free number and supplement telephone assistance with e-mail to facilitate student communication during hours the library is not open. After-hours reference service options (i.e., automated answering of frequently answered questions and automated fax-back services for delivery of library user guides) also can be used.

DE students, many of whom have conflicting family and work responsibilities, often work on course work during nights and weekends. Thus, they need access to library support services during this time. Although support can be provided using after-hours response options, students working on assignments during these times need quick turnaround times on requested information (interlibrary loans sometimes require an answer from a "live" person before the next workday when their assignment is due).

One approach to assuring that students have access to learning resources is to place articles, reprints of book chapters, or diagrams in a course handbook that students can order through the mail. There are services that will obtain copyright clearance for these resources. Students prefer having required readings readily accessible and are willing to pay for the convenience of having a packet of required course resources. Another approach is to place all assigned readings on electronic reserve in the library or on the course site on the Web-based learning management system. Electronic reserve would allow students enrolled in the course to have computer access to the assigned readings. However, 80% to 90% of library materials remain available only in print format because of copyright issues and cost. Thus, it is still necessary to support delivery of print materials to students as well as providing access to electronic reserves (Butler, 1997).

Library support has changed dramatically in the last 10 years as technology has been incorporated throughout the provision of services (Rodman, 2001). An excellent information resource regarding library support of DE initiatives is available at http://alexia.list.uiuc.edu/~b-sloan/libdist.htm. Guidelines on distance education library services have also been published by the Association of College and Research Libraries. Although the provision of services will vary from institution to institution, these resources serve as guidelines for the improvement of current services and the development of new services.

Bookstore Access

The campus bookstore should arrange for DE students to obtain the necessary textbooks. Bookstore staff can make up a list of required textbooks that are accessible via the Web or can be mailed to students. Student ordering of textbooks could be handled via the Web or mail and books shipped to students prior to the beginning of the semester. Bookstore personnel should be available to answer questions and to assist students during expanded hours prior to the beginning of the semester, to serve the needs of working students and students from different geographic locations.

SOCIAL SPACES

Teaching and learning are social activities, and faculty and students have an experience base in traditional and face-to-face educational settings where social spaces are well defined and assumed. In DE, however, the opportunity for interaction, social and intellectual discourse, and use of nonverbal cues changes dramatically. Faculty and students must establish different types of social spaces in order to overcome the barriers imposed by distance.

Facilitating Student Interaction

Establishing a sense of community in DE courses is necessary to overcome the barriers of distance and technology and, in some instances, lack of visual cues. Cobb and Mueller (1998) found that some students had a sense of isolation from peers and faculty when enrolled in a Web-based course. Students enrolled in videoconference-based DE can be assisted to overcome the perception of isolation by allowing time for student and faculty interaction via videoconference before and after class for questions and to provide an opportunity for networking. Virtual cafés and unmonitored chats can be set up for students enrolled in Web-based courses. Cobb and Mueller found that students enrolled in Web-based courses were overwhelmed about the high volume of messages on the course bulletin board. If personal chit-chat is found to contribute to this high message volume, a separate bulletin board for personal interaction can be established to redirect the flow of such messages.

Facilitating Faculty Interaction

Interaction with faculty inside and outside the course goes to the heart of education and is critical to learning (Anderson & Garrison, 1998). Recent work using computer-mediated collaboration tools indicates that cognitive apprenticeship models—socially interactive relationships between novices and experts to socialize students into a profession—evolve as students have increased interaction with the faculty (Bonk & Cunningham, 1998). Regular office hours also must be established to decrease students' perception of isolation from faculty. By using computer-mediated collaboration tools, faculty access can be more direct. Office hours in a chat group or using a toll-free number can provide time for formal and informal discussion with faculty.

Students are frustrated by changes in communication imposed by technology. Cobb and Mueller (1998) found that students perceived communication via the Web as impersonal in nature. They reported their greatest barrier was not seeing an instructor face-to-face. Providing some course materials via videotape, CD-ROM, or DVD provides an opportunity for students to have a visual connection with instructors. Shutte (1997) also found that students in a virtual classroom seemed frustrated by their inability to ask the professor questions in person. If faculty have a camera attached to their computer software, such as NetMeeting, this will support transmission of images as well as voices. This visual enhancement is important to some students and may provide more of a feeling of meeting with the professor in person and enhances students' feelings of connectedness with instructors (Oehlkers & Gibson, 2001).

ASSISTING STUDENTS TO DEVELOP PERSONAL AND STUDY SUPPORT SYSTEMS

Students who are learning alone require additional personal and academic support to overcome the isolation imposed by DE. Faculty can assist students to be aware of these needs, embed strategies for student support within the course, and provide suggestions for obtaining additional resources as needed.

Personal Support

One little-appreciated resource in DE courses is the support families and employers can provide. This support may be even more important than that provided by peers and faculty, and it affects students' persistence (Oehlkers, 1998). Pym (1992) found that family support is essential to student success in DE courses; it is also true that the family must understand the importance for "study time" on the Internet and be supportive to the student who is "in class" while at home. Billings (1988) found that in correspondence courses (which may have similarities to the isolation of Internet courses) students relied on family and employer support to overcome barriers of isolation. Other strategies can be used to assist learners in overcoming the barriers of DE technology, such as establishing outreach sites where face-to-face assistance is available if needed. Another strategy is to identify several students within the course who have used the technology in previous courses and ask them to be available to serve as peer "technology tutors," or employ a student who is adept with the technology to assist as needed.

The workplace can be an important source of support. Students should be encouraged to talk with coworkers about their learning and also to discuss learning issues applicable to their work situation in the DE classroom. Students reported that when coworkers were aware they were taking classes, the coworkers asked how the classes were going and volunteered to switch shifts near the time when papers were due and exams were scheduled (Oehlkers, 1998). Oehlkers also found that some employers provided tuition assistance, whereas supervisors were sabotaging students with work schedules that conflicted with their courses. He suggests that educators collaborate with employers for mutual benefit and learner support.

Course Study Support

Another type of support that students may need is assistance with the course content and in learning the content and skills of the course. Course tutors may be assigned to courses where students can be anticipated to have difficulty. Course tutors can be students from a previous course, a teaching assistant with the content knowledge of the course, or nurses in the community who can serve as study mentors. These supports may be based at a learning outreach center, collaborative campus site, or clinical agency, or through the use of the technology the tutor may have time on air or within the Web-based courses. The role of the tutor may vary from course to course and can involve assisting students to learn the content of the course and to develop writing or math skills or serving as a role model. Having study tutors in DE courses is particularly important if course completion rates have been low, if students have difficulty with course concepts, or if they do not have well-developed prerequisite course skills such as language proficiency.

Peer study groups are another support for students. These groups may form spontaneously or with direction from the course faculty. Study groups can form at outreach centers or employment settings when a cohort of students is enrolled in a program. In televised courses, faculty can allocate time for small groups to work together. The Internet offers faculty an easy way for students to work together by using e-mail or a separate chat room or bulletin board established for this purpose within a Web-based course.

ESTABLISHING A STUDENT-CENTERED DISTANCE-EDUCATION LEARNING COMMUNITY

The ultimate support for the learner is a course designed to encourage learning by taking advantage of the particular distance-delivery technology, as well as faculty who are prepared to serve as guides, coaches, learning mentors, and facilitators. Although there are specific course design and implementation strategies unique to each DE delivery system

(Billings & Bachmeier, 1994; Harasim et al., 1996), years of research in teaching and learning have revealed seven principles of good education (active learning, respect for diverse talents and ways of learning, rich and rapid feedback, interaction and collaboration with peers, interaction with faculty, time on task, and high expectations), which when used consistently lead to effective learning outcomes and student satisfaction (Chickering & Gamson, 1987). These principles also are effective when used in technology-mediated courses (Chickering & Ehrmann, 1996) and can serve as a framework for choosing teaching-learning activities that guide students in achieving learning outcomes and personal goals.

High expectations are set through clearly defined course goals and objectives and negotiation of learning contracts within the course (Porter, 1997). Students in DE achieve learning outcomes as well as do students in traditional on-campus courses that use face-to-face instruction (Billings & Bachmeier, 1994).

Prompt feedback about the learning process, as well as outcomes, guides students toward learning goals and overcomes a sense of isolation. Additional feedback can be requested and provided by faculty, classmates, peers, professional colleagues, and experts. Faculty can support student learning by anticipating points in the course where students may require additional feedback and design activities to give feedback as needed. Though prompt feedback is certainly an educational support issue, there is an emotional support component as well. Mueller (2001) found that when sending files digitally to faculty, students worried about whether their file reached the faculty member if an acknowledgment of receipt was not provided. Faculty should either post an announcement on the learning management system or send an e-mail to students acknowledging receipt of digital assignments to minimize students' worries that their files may have disappeared into a great black hole.

Electronic collaboration tools can be used in DE classes to promote increased interaction with classmates (Bonk & Cunningham, 1998; Harasim, 1993). These tools promote group work, enhanced communication among class members, and formation of peer support groups. In fact, one of the advantages of DE courses is the richness of students with a variety of experiences and viewpoints. Faculty can encourage and guide this interaction to facilitate learning outcomes.

Active learning occurs when members of the learning community are socially and cognitively engaged in the course. Active learning aids comprehension and retention of course content, and faculty can design course activities that engage students with content and each other. Active learning is promoted through authentic learning experiences, by solving real problems, using problem-based learning, and developing meaningful products. Embedding these experiences in DE courses leads to relevant learning outcomes and contributions to the knowledge in the profession.

Respect for diversity is demonstrated by providing different ways of attaining learning outcomes, creating a climate in which there is respect for different cultures and viewpoints, and providing options for using a variety of learning styles. Faculty can facilitate this respect and model it through course design and implementation.

WHAT DISTANCE EDUCATION IS LIKE FOR STUDENTS

Being a member of a DE learning community requires changes in approaches to learning on the part of the student and additional services for technical, academic, personal, and career support on the part of the institution providing the educational offering. The learning support services suggested have been shown to provide a more positive outcome for students and to facilitate their transition to these new modes of education. Common problems noted during transition include student satisfaction levels, frustration with technology, feelings of isolation, and perception of increased time spent on coursework. However, the better the student support, the smoother the transition for students and the more positive the experience. This results in increased student satisfaction and increased student retention.

Swan (1999) found that students taking courses via interactive video-conference systems were generally satisfied with the quality of instruction and believed that it was a good method for offering courses. However, when asked about the negative points of courses via videoconference, they responded that it was boring to stare at a television screen for the entire class period, that they were unable to see everyone at once, and that sending papers away to be graded was problematic. Swan also noted that students reported a perception that all remote sites did not get the same amount of attention. Wuest (1989) noted that there was increased participation and therefore increased attention to students at the studio site of an audio-teleconference class.

Students in DE courses identify communication with faculty as a problem and requested more frequent communication with faculty during the course, as well as prompt feedback on course assignments (Blakely & Curran-Smith, 1998; Reinert & Fryback, 1997; Sherwood, Armstrong, & Bond, 1994). Engaging students during DE has shown to be helpful in alleviating communication problems. Fulmer, Hazzard, Jones, and Keene (1992) noted that although students were initially uncomfortable participating in videoconference courses, encouragement facilitated participation. When interactive teaching strategies were used in an interactive videoconference class, students reported feeling closer to the faculty and to the school (Sherwood et al., 1994).

Students continue to identify frustrations with technological shortcomings of equipment used with distance education (Boyd & Baker, 1987; Cobb & Mueller, 1998; Phillips, Hagenbush, & Baldwin, 1992). However, despite these frustrations, most students indicated that they would take another course via DE.

Ridley, Bailey, Davies, Hash, and Varner (1997) found that students enrolled in online courses cited the ability to reduce the negative effects of distance and scheduling as reasons for enrolling in Internet courses. However, even students who had a positive experience with a doctoral course in a virtual classroom on the Internet preferred to come to campus if able to do so, despite the benefits of convenience and access with the Internet course (Milstead & Nelson, 1998).

Student attitudes toward DE vary in level of satisfaction from enjoyment to anger or dislike of DE courses. Cobb and Mueller (1998) surveyed graduate students who had taken a Web-based course and found both positive and negative attitudes. Students who enjoyed the Web-based courses stated that it was a wonderful learning tool. They commented that it made learning more accessible and reported that they liked the convenience of having class at home. Other students, however, expressed strong negative feelings regarding Web-based courses. Some of these students reported difficulty learning while using computers. Others expressed the belief that Internet courses were no more than correspondence courses. Several students complained that Internet courses only provided an opportunity for visual learning, and they reported difficulty in comprehending what they read on the computer. These frustrations were also noted by Schutte (1997) and Cragg (1994).

Careful attention to course design can help make Internet courses a good learning experience for students. Faculty should pay special attention to the number of learning activities that are scheduled and the time they take for completion. Internet courses require an adjustment in teaching style and pedagogy to maximize effective learning and ensure that course requirements can be completed in a timely manner. A number of continuing education offerings are available to introduce faculty to these changes in teaching pedagogy and help faculty to be effective in a "virtual classroom."

Cobb and Mueller (1998) found that students complained about the increased time commitment required for Internet courses. Students reported that "class discussion" via a bulletin board took a great deal of time, especially in classes with a large number of students. Students reported difficulty sorting through large numbers of bulletin board messages when they all were somewhat significant. Students in large classes found that they had to log on daily to keep up with content, an expectation for which they were not prepared.

The students' report that time spent on Web courses was greater than in a traditional classroom is supported by Schutte (1997), who found that students in a virtual classroom perceived that they spent significantly more time on course work than did students in a traditional classroom setting. Time constraints may be a particular problem for graduate nursing students because they are predominantly female. Von Prummer (1994) noted that females enrolled in education placed greater emphasis on their family roles, which created role and time conflicts, whereas male students reported no role conflicts and mentioned being relieved of family duties and given uninterrupted time and space for studying.

Students reported a perception of decreased interaction with faculty and other students (Cobb & Mueller, 1998). This is in contrast to Schutte (1997), who noted more involvement among peers in a virtual classroom. He found that the highest-performing students reported the most peer interaction; however, peer interaction was built into the assignments for students in the virtual classroom but not for students in the traditional classroom. Cragg (1994) reported that computer conferencing allowed students to participate in discussions and schedule their own learning time. The group of students observed formed a cohesive, friendly group despite initial frustrations with the equipment. Campbell (1998) noted that women may have needs for support that differ from those of men because women more frequently talk about discomfort with isolation and place a higher value on connecting with others than men do. Because of these differences, faculty must remain vigilant for difficulties with peer interaction in computer-mediated courses.

Cobb and Mueller (1998) found that this decreased interaction also affected perceptions of faculty accessibility. Students reported that despite 24-hour, 7-day access to faculty via e-mail and the course bulletin board, it was very inconvenient, if not difficult, to seek help with problems. They were frustrated by having to wait until the next day (or week) for help. They identified that being unable to get immediate feedback on assignments or questions was a barrier; they wanted immediate input to know if they were on the right track.

SUMMARY

Technological advances in DE have provided a variety of delivery modes to increase access to nursing education. However, additional services are required to deliver effective DE to students and to assist students through the transition to these new modes of course delivery. Faculty who develop and teach DE courses must consider the need for these support systems, services, and resources prior to implementation of DE programs and monitor them for effectiveness. The student services support staff are truly the glue that holds DE programs together, and they influence student satisfaction and retention. Continued attention must be focused on what constitutes effective strategies for assuring the resources to support learner success.

REFERENCES

Anderson, L. P., Banks, S. R., & Leary, P. A. (2002). The effect of interactive television courses on student satisfaction. *Journal of Education for Business, 77,* 164–168.

Anderson, T. D., & Garrison, D. R. (1998). Learning in a networked world: New roles and responsibilities. In C. C. Gibson (Ed.), *Distance learners in higher education: Institutional responses for quality outcomes* (pp. 97–112). Madison, WI: Atwood.

Bedore, G. L., Bedore, M. R., & Bedore, G. L. (1998). *Online education: The future is now.* Phoenix, AZ: Art Press.

Billings, D. (1988). Attrition from correspondence courses: Development and testing a model of course completion. *Continuing Higher Education Review, 52*(3), 141–154.

Billings, D. M., & Bachmeier, B. (1994). Teaching and learning at a distance: A review of the literature. In L. R. Allen (Ed.), *Review of research in nursing education* (pp. 1–32). New York: National League for Nursing.

Blakely, J. A., & Curran-Smith, J. (1998). Teaching and community health nursing by distance methods: Development, process, and evaluation. *Journal of Continuing Education in Nursing, 29*(4), 148–153.

Bonk, C. J., & Cunningham, D. J. (1998). Searching for learner-centered, constructivist, and sociocultural components of collaborative educational learning tools. In C. J. Bonk & K. S. King (Eds.), *Electronic collaborators* (pp. 25–50). Mahwah, NJ: Erlbaum.

Boyd, S., & Baker, C. M. (1987). Using television to teach. *Nursing and Health Care, 8,* 523–528.

Brindley, J. E., von Ossietzky, C., & Paul, R. H. (2004). The role of learner support of transformation. Retrieved from http://www.change.co.nz/docs/eden/Brindley.pdf

Butler, J. (1997). *From the margins to the mainstream: Developing library support for distance learning.* Retrieved from http://www.lib.umn.edu/pubs/LibLine/LLvol8no4.html

Campbell, K. (1998). The Web: Design for active learning. Retrieved from http://www.alt.ualberta.ca/presentations/learnchar/learnchar.html

Cartwright, J. C., & Menkens, R. (2002). Student perspectives on transitioning to new technologies for distance learning. *Computers in Nursing, 20*(4), 143–149.

Chickering, A. W., & Ehrmann, S. (1996). Implementing the seven principles: Technology as lever. Retrieved from http://www.titlgroup.org/ehrmann.htm

Chickering, A. W., & Gamson, Z. F. (1987, October). Seven principles for good practice in undergraduate education. *AAHE Bulletin,* (3), 3–6.

Cobb, K. L., & Mueller, C. L. (1998). *Evaluation of graduate students in a virtual classroom.* Unpublished manuscript.

Cragg, C. E. (1994). Distance learning through computer conferences. *Nurse Educator, 19*(2), 10–14.

DeBourgh, G. A. (2003). Predictors of student satisfaction in distance delivered graduate nursing courses: What matters most? *Journal of Professional Nursing, 19,* 149–163.

Farrell, G. (2001). The changing faces of virtual education. Retrieved from http://www.col.org/virtualed/

Fulmer, J., Hazzard, M., Jones, S., & Keene, K. (1992). Distance learning: An innovative approach to nursing education. *Journal of Professional Nursing, 8,* 289–294.

Garrison, D. R., & Baynton, M. (1987). Beyond independence in distance education: Concept of control. *American Journal of Distance Education, 1*(3), 3–15.

Granger, D. (1989). Supporting individual learners at a distance. Proceedings of the Helping Learners at a Distance 5th Annual Conference on Teaching at a Distance (pp. 82–86). Madison: University of Wisconsin.

Harasim, L. (1993). Collaborating in cyberspace: Using computer conferencing as a group environment. *Interactive Learning Environments, 3*(2), 119–130.

Harasim, L., Hiltz, S. R., Teles, L., & Turoff, M. (1996). *Learning networks: A field guide to teaching and learning online.* Cambridge, MA: MIT Press.

Henry, P. (1993). Distance learning through audioconferencing. *Nurse Educator, 18*(2), 23–26.

Kazmer, M. M. (2002). Distance education students speak to the library: Here's how you can help even more. *The Electronic Library, 20,* 395–400.

Milstead, J. A., & Nelson, R. (1998). Preparation of an online asychronous university doctoral course: Lessons learned. *Computers in Nursing, 16,* 247–258.

Mueller, C. L. (2001). *Master of science in nursing students' experiences as members of a virtual classroom on the Internet.* Unpublished doctoral dissertation.

Oehlkers, R. (1998). Focus: Informal support. *Distance Education Systemwide Interactive Electronic Newsletter, 3*(9), 1–3.

Oehlkers, R. A., & Gibson, C. C. (2001). Learner support experienced by RNs in a collaborative distance RN-to-BSN program. *Journal of Continuing Education in Nursing, 32,* 266–273.

Phillips, C. Y., Hagenbush, E. G., & Baldwin, P. J. (1992). A collaborative effort in using telecommunications to enhance learning. *Journal of Continuing Education in Nursing, 23*(3), 134–138.

Phillips, M., & Kelly, P. (2001). Learning technologies for learner services. In E. J. Burge (Ed.), *The strategic use of learning technologies: New directions for adult and continuing education* (pp. 17–26). San Francisco: Jossey-Bass.

Porter, L. R. (1997). *Creating the virtual classroom: Distance learning with the Internet.* New York: Wiley.

Potter, J. (1998). Beyond access: Student perspectives on support service needs in distance education. *Canadian Journal of University Continuing Education, 24*(1), 59–82.

Pym, F. R. (1992). Women and distance education: A nursing perspective. *Journal of Advanced Nursing, 17,* 383–389.

Reinert, B., & Fryback, P. (1997). Distance learning and nursing education. *Journal of Nursing Education, 36,* 421–427.

Ridley, D. R., Bailey, B. L., Davies, E. S., Hash, S. G., & Varner, D. A. (1997, May). *Evaluating the impact of online course enrollments on FTEs at an urban university.* Paper presented at the annual forum of the Association for Institutional Research, Orlando, FL. (ERIC Document Reproduction Service No. ED410871)

Robinson, B. (1981). Support for student learning. In A. Kay & G. Rumble (Eds). *Distance teaching for higher and adult education* (pp. 141–161). London: Croom Helm.

Rodman, R. L. (2001). The S.A.G.E. project: A model for library support. *Internet Reference Services Quarterly, 6*(2), 35–45.

Rossiter, D., & Watters, J. (2000). *Technological literacy: Foundations for the 21st century.* Brisbane, Australia: Queensland University of Technology.

Schlossberg, N. K. (1984). *Counseling adults in transition.* New York: Springer.

Schutte, J. G. (1997). *Virtual teaching in higher education: The new intellectual superhighway or just another traffic jam?* Retrieved from http://www.csun.edu/sociology/virexp.htm

Sherwood, G. D., Armstrong, M. L., & Bond, M. L. (1994). Distance education programs: Defining issues of assessment, accessibility, and accommodation. *Journal of Continuing Education in Nursing, 25,* 251–257.

Stoffel, J. A. (1987). Meeting the needs of distance students: Feedback, support and promptness. *Lifelong Learning: Omnibus of Practice and Research, 11*(3), 25–28.

Swan, M. K. (1999). *Effectiveness of distance learning courses: Students' perceptions.* Retrieved from http://www.ssu.missouri.edu/SSU/AgEd/NAERM/s-a-4.htm

Von Prummer, C. (1994). Women-friendly perspectives in distance education. *Open Learning, 9*(1), 3–12.

Wuest, J. (1989). Debate: A strategy for increasing interaction in audioteleconferencing. *Journal of Advanced Nursing, 14,* 847–852.

CHAPTER 4

Faculty Preparation for Teaching Online

Arlene E. Johnson

Having moved into the twenty-first century, the impact of technology on teaching and learning has been significant. Many institutions of higher learning have embraced online learning as an answer to meeting the needs of today's students. The introduction of online learning into nursing education has resulted in a change in the role of the nurse educator. Many faculty are struggling with the paradigm shift toward online learning. This chapter will address many of the issues that are of concern to faculty who teach online.

COMPETENCIES NECESSARY TO TEACH ONLINE

One of the most critical issues that arises in the shift from traditional instruction to online instruction is the faculty's preparedness to teach online. Most faculty find the transition a difficult experience. Lack of technology knowledge is often identified as a significant barrier. Research indicates that lack of knowledge of the pedagogy related to online learning is a much greater problem (Conrad, 2004). Technology and pedagogy cannot be separated. There is a dynamic relationship among content, pedagogy, and technology (Koehler, Mishra, Hershey, & Peruski, 2004). The Higher Learning Commission, a commission of the North Central Association of Colleges and Schools, developed *Best Practices for Electronically Offered Degree and Certificate Programs (2000)* in response to the rapid growth of technologically mediated instruction in institutions of higher learning (North Central, 2000). The *Best Practices* document was created to present a consistent approach to the evaluation of distance education. The recommendations presented in the document focus on maintaining a balance between accountability and innovation.

Technology

Faculty members who teach online must acquire specialized skills. When faculty are given the assignment to teach online, many are concerned with their level of technological expertise. If a faculty member plans to convert a traditional classroom course to online, the ideal course conversion team would include the course instructor and an instructional designer. Once a course has been designed, the level of technology knowledge needed to teach an online course is quite basic. The basic technology competencies necessary to teach online are the abilities to (a) set up folders and directories; (b) use word processing software (cut, copy, paste, save files); (c) handle e-mail communications, including attachments; and (d) use a browser to access the World Wide Web (Ko & Rossen, 2004). It is also very important for faculty to become familiar with the technology support staff at their institutions.

If the course instructor is not able to collaborate with an instructional designer for course conversion, it will be necessary for the faculty member to use one of the online course delivery platforms (also known as course management systems), such as WebCT, Blackboard, or Educator to adapt the course materials into a format that can be accessed via the Web. An institution's technology department usually makes the decision about which course delivery platform will be used for all of its online courses. Many of the platforms have built-in Web authoring tools that allow the faculty to create Web pages without the need to know HTML (hypertext markup language). These tools are "pedagogically advanced platforms," which provide a variety of synchronous and asynchronous tools that can be used in teaching an online course (Moore, Winograd, & Lange, 2001). Included in many of the platforms are mechanisms for online testing and evaluation, as well the capability to track the progress of students. Faculty will need instruction and assistance in learning how to use the course delivery platform to convert instructional materials.

Instructor to Facilitator

The transition to the online classroom results in changes in the faculty and student roles. Instructors who feel confident in the face-to-face classroom may experience feelings of inadequacy or nervousness when teaching online. A lack of social cues can lead to misunderstandings or behaviors that might not occur when people are in a face-to-face environment. The anonymity that the online classroom provides gives some learners the opportunity to behave more aggressively than normal. Students who are strong in confidence in a traditional classroom may find themselves intimidated in the online environment. The more introverted student may actually flourish in the online classroom.

The online environment diffuses authority and places the student at the center of the learning process (Alexander, Polyakova-Norwood, Johnston, Christensen, & Loquist, 2003). Faculty-student relationships change. Some instructors report that they have experienced stronger relationships with students in the online environment, while others report feeling more distant (Ryan, Carlton, & Ali, 2004). The instructor's role in the online classroom is transformed from knowledge deliverer to facilitator, and students assume a greater responsibility for the learning that takes place. In online learning there is a shift in emphasis from course completion to competency-based education. There needs to be a balance of content delivery and the learners' need for a socially constructed environment. To achieve this, it is necessary for the instructor to relinquish a certain amount of control over the learning process. Often, faculty rely on their experience in the face-to-face classroom and find it difficult to let go of some of the old paradigm. Faculty have reported a role change from one of expert teacher in the classroom to that of a novice in the online classroom (Ryan et al., 2004).

Community Building

Students in online courses have reported feeling isolated and missing social contact with the instructor and peers (Attack & Rankin, 2002). In order for the learning process in the electronic classroom to be successful, attention needs to be paid to the developing sense of community within the group of participants. The learning community becomes the vehicle through which learning occurs (Palloff & Pratt, 1999). A dynamic community model supports an environment that promotes inquiry and supports learning. Most students bring prior experience and learning to the online classroom, which can contribute to the classroom learning success. Students must feel comfortable and willing to share these experiences

(Keeton, 2004). Helping students to become comfortable expressing their thoughts and feelings in writing is key to a successful online environment. To create a social presence in the online classroom, the instructor can model inclusion of feelings in written communications. When an instructor is successful in fostering community, students report they have a better learning experience, feel closer to their peers, and get to know their instructors better than they ever did in a traditional classroom (Lynch, 2002).

Faculty need to incorporate learning strategies that result in meaningful interactions between students and instructors. Moore (1989) identified a model that includes three types of interaction in the online classroom: learner-instructor interaction, learner-content interaction, and learner-learner interaction. Learner-instructor interaction is highly desired by learners. During learner-instructor interaction, the instructor should seek to stimulate the learners' interest in the course content, as well as encourage self-direction and self-motivation. Learner-content interaction is the process of the learner intellectually interacting with content that results in changes in the cognitive structures of the learner's mind. Learner-learner interaction occurs with or without the presence of the instructor, and can take place between two learners or within a group of learners. Collaborative learning activities allow learners to achieve a deeper level of knowledge generation. The most powerful experiences may be those in which interaction occurs throughout the group instead of between one participant and facilitator in a group setting (Palloff & Pratt, 1999).

ASSESSMENT OF STUDENT LEARNING

The design of an online course should emphasize an active learning environment with real-world application and knowledge construction through collaboration and problem-based learning. Assessment is an equally important part of the design of the course. Sound assessment strategy is not limited to a single measurement, but consists of multiple measurements that include diverse assessment tasks. No single assessment can ascertain whether all learning objectives have been achieved. A variety of assessment tasks are needed to provide a well-rounded view of learner progress (Rovai, 2000).

The shift in responsibility for learning from instructor to student in the online learning environment has resulted in a more competency-based model of assessment of student learning. Palloff and Pratt (2003) suggested that we need to develop a means to evaluate outcomes that is specific to online learning. Evaluation that is congruent with course learning objectives and is consistent with the learning activities in the course will likely result in an accurate assessment of student mastery of course concepts. Inclusion of self-assessment activities encourages students to reflect on the learning that has taken place.

Student assessment serves two purposes: to evaluate students' progress and to facilitate student learning. There must be a direct relationship between learning objectives and assessment measures. The following strategies can be used to develop this connection:

1. Obtain a good match between the type of objective you wish to measure (e.g., knowledge, skills, and attitudes) and the means you use to measure it.

2. Use several data sources to gain as complete a picture as possible.

3. Remember that not all instructional objectives lend themselves to direct, precise measurement. (Lynch, 2002, p. 118)

According to Robles and Braathen (2002), online assessment must be used to measure both learning objectives and students' application of knowledge. Assessment techniques should reflect the pedagogy of online courses. They identified three key components of assessment of student learning: "(a) measurements of the learning objectives, (b) self-assessments for students to measure their own achievement, and (c) interaction and feedback between and among the instructor and students" (p. 40). Robles and Braathen further stated that effective assessment must be active and authentic in the online environment. Students should be able to see the fit between the content of the course and real-world application.

FACULTY PERCEPTIONS OF TEACHING ONLINE

Nursing faculty teaching Web-based courses have a variety of perceptions of teaching online. Ryan et al. (2004) investigated the experiences of nursing faculty teaching Web-based courses. The faculty discussed perceptions of teaching online. Participants in this study agreed that an infrastructure is needed to ensure faculty success in teaching online. Administrative support is needed, as well as technical support. Faculty development is essential, including collaboration with experts in computer technology. Faculty who teach online benefit through sharing of experiences and ideas with other faculty. All of the participants in this study agreed that workload is heavier when teaching online courses. Policies should be developed to limit enrollments. It has been suggested that 20 to 30 students is a maximum number.

Benefits of Teaching Online

Faculty who teach online identify a number of benefits. One of the most important benefits is the time devoted to learning about online education, which results in a more student-centered approach to teaching and learning. Faculty who teach online also become comfortable with technology skills. It has also been reported that faculty get to know their students better, because of increased interaction in the online environment. Finally, faculty report that data obtained from their online teaching experiences provides them with additional opportunities for scholarship, such as presenting at conferences and publishing in peer-reviewed journals (Oakley, 2004).

Motivating Factors

The rapidly growing number of distance education programs has led researchers to explore faculty attitudes and motivating factors. There are differences in faculty attitudes by gender, faculty rank, and tenure status. Faculty who participate in distance education appear to be more highly motivated than nonparticipators are by intrinsic values, such as intellectual challenge and overall job satisfaction. Nonparticipating faculty appear to be more affected by personal needs (release time, credit toward promotion and tenure, and merit pay) and extrinsic motives (expectation by university, requirement by department, lack of technical background). Administrators identify factors associated with personal needs (reduced teaching load, release time, and monetary support for participation) higher than both groups of faculty. These findings indicate that there is a discrepancy between administrators' and faculty's perceptions on motivating factors for teaching online (Schifter, 2002).

In a review of the literature, Clay (1999) identified these factors that facilitate the willingness of faculty to embrace distance education:

1. The opportunity to reach remote students
2. Intellectual challenge and the opportunity to develop new ideas
3. The opportunity to work with students who are more motivated
4. Release time
5. Financial reward
6. Opportunities for research
7. Motivation to use technology
8. The opportunity for recognition

9. The opportunity to use support services
10. Reduced travel
11. Increased course quality
12. Increased flexibility

Resistors

Many individuals in higher education view change as threatening. Faculty members may have preconceived attitudes about technology and distance learning, which can be a barrier to adoption of online learning. From her review of the literature, Clay (1999) identified these primary factors inhibiting faculty from distance teaching:

1. Increased workload
2. The altered role of the instructor
3. Lack of technical and administrative support
4. Reduced course quality
5. Negative attitudes of colleagues

Those who have learned successful teaching/learning strategies without the use of technology question its relevance and therefore are reluctant to take on the challenge of technology-assisted instruction. Many faculty do not find value in learning the technology needed to teach online, as it takes time away from other responsibilities, which they view as more important. Institutions often lack faculty who have experience teaching online and could act as role models for less experienced faculty (Koehler et al., 2004).

It has been suggested that the social distance between instructors and their students is another barrier for faculty who are reluctant to teach in the online environment. The instructor can reduce the distance between teacher and student by engaging in frequent communication. E-mail is the most common form of one-on-one communication. However, students have identified that the online presence of the instructor matters most (Brooks, 2003). It is important for the instructor to be present in online discussions, while maintaining the role of facilitator and not overdirecting the discussion.

Development and Preparation Time

As the number of course offerings taught online in higher education has increased, so has discussion regarding additional responsibilities of faculty who teach these courses. Pachnowski and Jurczyk (2003) measured the effect that teaching in a distance learning environment had on a faculty's time and teaching and the impact that teaching in that environment should have on load policy and reward. All of the participants reported that they had extra preparation time (due to technology) to prepare for a semester course. Fifty percent of the teachers reported that they spent more than 30 hours in preparation for the first semester they taught the course. The data showed that as faculty members progressed through each semester, they required less preparation time beyond what would be expected from a traditional classroom course. There were still one third of faculty who required a significant amount of preparation time in the second, third, or fourth time teaching a Web-based course. The amount of technology training required by faculty decreased each semester. The results of this study indicate that faculty who engage in Web-based teaching may require some accommodations during the first semester that a course is taught, due to the additional time it takes to prepare the course for conversion to online. Administrators could use the data from this study to develop faculty load policies that would provide additional preparation time for faculty during the initial semesters of teaching a distance course.

COMPENSATION AND WORKLOAD

Concerns about faculty workload have been a reported deterrent to participation in online teaching. There is a perception that online courses require more development and preparation time for the instructor, compared with traditional classroom instruction. This has not been consistently documented in the literature related to online learning. Some faculty find that the time spent teaching online is not actually greater, but the "chunking" or flow of tasks online is different, which results in a sense that less productive time is available for other teaching responsibilities. For example, the expectation that faculty members reply to student messages several times daily means that the uninterrupted time necessary for research and other scholarly works no longer exists. It is important for faculty to identify strategies that could be used to decrease workload in online courses (Thompson, 2004).

A 1997 survey conducted by the RAND Institute (as cited in Palloff & Pratt, 1999) indicated that courses delivered online can actually decrease central administrative costs while reaching out to students who otherwise may not have had access to the university. Although on-campus resources may be saved, there are the additional costs of technology, transmission, maintenance, and technical support. The idea that the larger the class, the greater the return does not apply to the electronic classroom. Palloff and Pratt wrote that it is essential to limit class size when delivering courses online. They proposed that given the lower costs involved in delivery, class sizes can be kept small without reducing revenue. These authors also addressed the issue of course fees. Many universities charge the same fees for face-to-face and online learners. Online learners sometimes complain about this, because they do not see the direct costs involved with online learning. Students who learn in this environment need to see a high degree of involvement by faculty and technical support. Providing online learning may not be less expensive for institutions.

Even though the total time commitment in teaching online courses may fall within reasonable expectations, the instructor needs to be online and available to students each day, unlike live courses that meet between one and three times a week. Participating in and grading online discussions takes the greatest amount of time, but the discussions show that the students post four to five times as many messages as the instructor does. Students have more opportunities to respond to and interact in online courses than they do in traditional lecture courses (Lazarus, 2003). Students in online courses expect faculty to be more readily and promptly available in responding to student's communications (Keeton, 2004).

Compensation and workload policies are needed to address the additional time it takes for faculty to develop and teach online courses. Even though a number of studies have shown that faculty who choose to teach online do so for personal or intrinsic rewards rather than monetary rewards, adequate compensation is needed to support and retain faculty who have agreed to take on this challenge.

Promotion and Tenure

Faculty have found that the traditional role comprised of teaching, scholarship, and service has been affected by the introduction of technology into the classroom. The promotion and tenure system in most institutions of higher learning values research and scholarly publication above other faculty activities. Tenure status and academic rank have an effect on the adoption of distance education (Jones, Linder, Murphy, & Dooley, 2002; Schifter, 2002). Faculty at the academic rank of instructor or assistant professor and nontenured are more comfortable and competent with technology needed to implement distance education (Jones et al., 2002). Faculty in these categories are often discouraged from participating in distance education, because of promotion and tenure concerns. Preparing for and teaching distance education is very time-consuming and it may take away from research time. Therefore, younger and less senior faculty may be reluctant to participate, due to potential implications of lack of time for research and other scholarly work. More experienced tenured faculty may benefit the most from training in the use of instructional technologies. Restructuring the promotion and tenure system may attract a wider range of faculty who will make the commitment to online learning.

LIBRARY SERVICES

Surveys on library usage indicate that library users, including distance learners, are interested in technology and the use of computers to pursue knowledge. As access to information through electronic means increases, the learning environment is becoming more technologically complex (Derlin & Erazo, 1997). The transition to technology-assisted instruction brings new challenges to library services. There is a debate on how much reliance there should be on printed media. How will electronic equipment be preserved in the case of system failure? How much space should be devoted to storing information (digital or physical)? The librarian's role in the future may be one of information specialist, who can provide guidance on use of library technology and access of information from various locations. Librarians will also collaborate with faculty to develop learning activities for distance learners. Copyright and fair use policies will be challenged and revised as technology continues to develop.

Faculty involved in online education report that finding information has become both easier and more difficult with the use of technology: easier because access to information across the world is now possible through a variety of search tools; more difficult because of the vast amount of information available on the Web. Faculty have a general lack of knowledge about electronic resources and services and the range of databases available to them (Jankowska, 2004).

INTELLECTUAL PROPERTY

Online learning has created many new questions about ownership and control of online materials. Faculty have concerns about the ability to edit and control the presentation of works they have created, as well as the ability to change and update the materials over time. They also have concerns about the ability to take educational materials they have created when they leave to work at another institution. Institutions have increasing concerns about online educational materials because of the financial and technical resources required to develop online courses. Many institutions have developed policies indicating that the institution owns copy-rightable works that are created with "substantial," "significant," or "extraordinary" university resources.

The best policies and practices of ownership and use of online course materials would recognize and balance the rights of the course creators and contributors with the needs of the institution (Alger, 2002). Many of the legal and policy standards in higher education are based on the traditional model of face-to-face instruction. The emergence of online learning has caused institutions of higher learning to reexamine policies related to curriculum development and control, evaluation of faculty and students, and ownership and use of intellectual property. One of the differences between traditional education and distance education is that individuals who create original online course materials may not necessar-ily be the instructor who teaches the course. The faculty member who created the course may not be at all involved in the use of the materials. The faculty who are responsible for delivery of the course content may not have the same expertise as the course creator. Alger raised these questions that arise in this type of arrangement:

- Who is responsible for revising the course?

- What happens if the course originator moves to another institution?

- Who makes the ultimate decision when conflicts arise among creators and instructors of courses?

- Who is responsible for ensuring compliance with copyright law in the use of course materials?

- What is the impact of fair use of offering such courses to non–degree-seeking students on a for-profit basis? (Alger, 2002, p. 5)

ACADEMIC INTEGRITY

The evaluation of students in online courses raises several important issues. Instructors must create safeguards to ensure that students are held to the same standards of academic integrity as students who learn in traditional classrooms. The key to ensuring academic rigor in online courses is to meet the learning objectives as the classroom counterpart (Lynch, 2002). The means to measure student mastery of course outcomes may have to be modified in the online environment. If there is no similar traditional course, it would be important to follow online instructional design principles. The course learning outcomes must be clearly identified and instructional activities that encourage active learning should be developed. Learning outcomes and strategies should be linked to methods that will be used to assess students' mastery of competencies.

The two most common issues of academic honesty in online learning are identity crisis and plagiarism. Identity crisis refers to the issue of how do we know the person online is the person who registered for the class? The identity problem is difficult to address, because the complex technology needed to identify an individual in a remote setting is very expensive. It would be prudent to create course activities and assessments that make it more difficult for students to cheat due to frequency of participation or application of theory to the students' own lives. There are software programs available that can be used to detect plagiarism, but these are time-consuming to use. The best prevention of plagiarism is student education and reinforcement throughout the course.

Proctored testing may be relevant for a summative assessment, such as an end of course exam. Proctored testing at decentralized locations is available to students at locations away from their own campuses. The Consortium of College Testing Centers (CCTC) is a free referral service provided by the National College Testing Association. CCTC consists of a group of college and university testing centers throughout the United States that provides proctored testing at decentralized locations. CCTC can be accessed at http://testing.byu.edu/NCTA/Consortium/. Safeguards should be built into the online course design that will require online learners to uphold the same standards of academic honesty as students in traditional courses. Careful design of summative assessments is another approach that could be used to assess student learning. Authentic performance assessments, such as projects that are relevant to the learner, may be a better assessment than a traditional essay test.

When planning for implementation of online programs, it is essential to gain the support and enthusiasm of the faculty. Those leading the initiative must assess the factors that will facilitate the change and those that will become barriers. Teaching online is not better or worse than face-to-face teaching. Both modes of instruction are unique, each with its own advantages and disadvantages. The two teaching methods can be used in the same course without compromising or denigrating the other. They can form a synergistic union that strengthens both (Glahn & Gen, 2002).

REFERENCES

Alexander, J. W., Polyakova-Norwood, V., Johnston, L. W., Christensen, P., & Loquist, R. S. (2003). Collaborative development and evaluation of an online nursing course [Electronic version]. *Distance Education, 24*(1), 41–56.

Alger, J. R. (2002). Online policy, ethics and law: What you need to know. Part I: Quality and integrity issues [Electronic version]. *Distance Education Report, 6*(11), 2, 6.

Attack, L., & Rankin, J. (2002). A descriptive study of registered nurses' experiences with web-based learning [Electronic version]. *Journal of Advanced Nursing, 40,* 457–4

Brooks, L. (2003). How the attitudes of instructors, students, course administrators, and course designers affect the quality of an online learning environment. *Online Journal of Distance Learning Administration, 6*(4). Retrieved May 19, 2004, from http://www.westga.edu/~distance/ojdla/winter64/brooks64.htm

Clay, M. (1999). Development of training and support programs for distance education instructors. *Online Journal of Distance Learning Administration, 2*(3). Retrieved August 26, 2004, from http://www.westga.edu/~distance/clay23.html

Conrad, D. (2004). University instructors' reflections on their first online teaching experiences [Electronic version]. *Journal of Asynchronous Learning Networks, 3*(1), 7–18.

Derlin, R. L., & Erazo, E. (1997). Distance learning and the digital library: Transforming the library into an information center. In T. E. Cyrs (Ed.), *Teaching and learning at a distance* (pp. 103–117). San Francisco: Jossey-Bass.

Glahn, R., & Gen, R. (2002). Progenies in education: The evolution of internet teaching [Electronic version]. *Community College Journal of Research and Practice, 26,* 777–785.

Jankowska, M. A. (2004). Identifying university professors' information needs in the challenging environment of information and communication technologies [Electronic version]. *Journal of Academic Librarianship, 30*(1), 51–66.

Jones, E. T., Linder, J. R., Murphy, T. H., & Dooley, K. E. (2002). Faculty philosophical position towards distance education: Competency, value, and educational technology support. *Online Journal of Distance Learning Administration, 5*(1). Retrieved June 3, 2003, from http://www.westga.edu/~distance/ojdla/spring51/jones51.html

Keeton, M. T. (2004). Best online instruction practices: Report of Phase I of an ongoing study [Electronic version]. *Journal of Asynchronous Learning Networks, 8*(2), 75–100.

Ko, S., & Rossen, S. (2004). *Teaching online: A practical guide* (2nd ed.). Boston: Houghton Mifflin.

Koehler, M. J., Mishra, P. A., Hershey, K., & Peruski, L. (2004). With a little help from your students: A new model for faculty development and online course design [Electronic version]. *Journal of Technology and Teacher Education, 12*(1), 25–55.

Lazarus, B. D. (2003). Teaching courses online: How much time does it take? [Electronic version]. *Journal of Asynchronous Learning Networks, 7*(3), 47–54.

Lynch, M. M. (2002). *The online educator: A guide to creating the virtual classroom.* London: Routledge Falmer.

Moore, G. S., Winograd, K., & Lange, D. (2001). *You can teach online: Building a creative learning environment.* New York: McGraw-Hill.

Moore, M. G. (1989). Three types of interaction. *American Journal of Distance Education, 3*(2). Retrieved August 26, 2004, from http://www.ajde.com/Contents/vol3_2.htm

North Central Association Commission on Institutions of Higher Education. (2000). *Guidelines for distance education.* Retrieved June 28, 2004, from http://www.ncacihe.org/resources/guidelines/gdistance.html

Oakley, B. (2004). The value of online learning: Perspectives from the University of Illinois at Springfield [Electronic version]. *Journal of Asynchronous Learning Networks, 8*(3), 22–32.

Pachnowski, L. M., & Jurczyk, J. P. (2003). Perceptions of faculty on the effect of distance learning technology on faculty preparation time. *Online Journal of Distance Learning Administration, 6*(3). Retrieved June 29, 2004, from http://www.westga.edu/~distance/ojdla/fall63/pachnowski64.html

Palloff, R. M., & Pratt, K. (1999). *Building learning communities in cyberspace: Effective strategies for the online classroom.* San Francisco: Jossey-Bass.

Palloff, R. M., & Pratt, K. (2003). *The virtual student: A profile and guide to working with online learners.* San Francisco: Jossey-Bass.

Robles, M., & Braathen, S. (2002). Online assessment techniques [Electronic version]. *Delta Pi Epsilon Journal, 14*(1), 39–49.

Rovai, A. P. (2000). Online and traditional assessments: What is the difference? [Electronic version]. *Internet and Higher Education, 3,* 141–151.

Ryan, M., Carlton, K., & Ali, N. S. (2004). Role of faculty in distance learning and changing pedagogies [Electronic version]. *Nursing Education Perspectives, 25*(2), 73–80.

Schifter, C. (2002). Perception differences about participating in distance education. *Online Journal of Distance Learning Administration, 5*(1). Retrieved June 3, 2003, from http://www.westga.edu/~distance/ojdla/spring51/schifter51.html

Thompson, M. M. (2004). Faculty self study research project: Examining the online workload [Electronic version]. *Journal of Asynchronous Learning Networks, 8*(3), 84–88.

CHAPTER 5

Using Clinical Simulations in Distance Education

Pamela R. Jeffries, Marcella T. Hovancsek, and
John M. Clochesy

AN OVERVIEW OF SIMULATIONS
IN NURSING EDUCATION

An important challenge of nurse educators is to develop efficient and effective methods to teach decision making, critical thinking, and problem-solving skills to an increasingly diverse population of students. In the past, educators believed it was enough to provide students with a variety of clinical experiences in which learners could apply the classroom content to become a competent nurse. Today, however, experienced nurses, staff development educators, and managers agree that many students and new graduates lack the critical thinking skills needed to work in increasingly complex clinical environments. To meet the diverse needs of students and graduates working in these complex environments, clinical simulations are being designed and implemented in nursing courses and programs. Providing simulations in nursing education is a relatively efficient method of teaching content and critical-thinking skills safely and in collaboration with the instructor without fear of causing harm to actual patients (Weis & Guyton-Simmons, 1998). This can be particularly helpful in distance education, where students are not physically present with the teacher to practice clinical techniques. This practice can be "simulated" through CD-ROMs, the Internet, or by use of a preceptor model. Using a preceptor model, an assigned responsible person can be accountable for teaching and evaluating the learners' skills in a physical environment while the student learns content in a distance learning platform (Billings et al., in press). In this chapter, advantages and challenges of using simulations, general concepts of using simulations, and how simulations are being used in distance education today will be described. Additional sections will discuss simulations used as (a) a teaching-learning intervention; (b) an enhancement to clinical practice; (c) an assessment method; and (d) a blended teaching-learning model when combined with distance education. Implications for the nurse educator related to these multiple uses will be discussed.

Incorporating simulations into the educational environment provides many advantages, but implementing simulation strategies can also challenge the educator. Table 5.1 lists the advantages and challenges of using simulations in the educational arena. Despite the challenges, however, this innovative, interactive educational strategy is being used increasingly in many different arenas of health care and other disciplines.

GENERAL CONCEPTS OF SIMULATIONS

Types of Simulations

Simulations are defined as events or situations made to resemble clinical practice as closely as possible (Seropian, 2003). Various types of simulations are being incorporated into the teaching-learning environment today. Full-scale patient simulations using high-fidelity, sophisticated patient simulators provide a high level of interactivity and realism to the learner. Less sophisticated, but still educationally useful, other simulators involve the use of computer-based simulations in which the participant relies on a two-dimensional focused experience to problem solve, perform a skill, or make decisions during the clinical scenario. Studies have shown the two-dimensional experience has merit in terms of positive learning outcomes and skill acquisition (Jeffries, Woolf, & Linde, 2003). Part-task training devices, such as IV arms and haptic (forced feedback) IV trainers are used in simulations for psychomotor skills with the learner able to practice a skill repeatedly before performing it on a real patient. The part-task trainers typically ensure a satisfactory rate of achievement of objectives and benefit to the participant. Studies have shown that these

TABLE 5.1 Advantages and Challenges of Using Simulations in Nursing

Advantages: Simulations provide	Challenges: Simulations may
1. a safe, nonthreatening environment to practice skills and decision making	1. increase faculty preparation time
2. a strategy to promote active learning	2. require more physical space than available
3. a standardized learning situation where all participants can obtain the experience	3. involves greater expense, i.e., equipment, personnel, and other resources
4. a controlled learning environment	4. change the focus of teaching from teacher-centered to student-centered
5. a mechanism to enhance psychomotor skills	5. increase learner anxiety
6. a strategy to provide collaborative team work that can be practiced and evaluated	6. limit the number of students that can participate at once
7. a mechanism to provide planned learning time for the learner or participant	7. require computer literacy and technical support, if the simulation is computer-based or a patient simulator
8. an opportunity for immediate feedback and discussion over the case scenario	
9. an opportunity to practice managing rare or infrequent events	

task trainers do instruct the participants on the psychomotor skill and that the skill set is transferred to the real-patient environment (Engum & Jeffries, 2003; Hovancsek, Horn, Jamison, & Narsavage, 2004). Programs or courses in which the task-trainers are used include clinical laboratory courses and modules during which specific skill sets and goals need to be obtained. From a distance-learning environment, the course content can be learned from the Web-based course, with the actual skill being assigned to be performed in the laboratory on a task trainer with a preceptor facilitating the experience. Two-dimensional CD ROMs can also provide interactive practice with skills if simulators are not available.

The Instructor's Role

Teachers are essential to the success of using interactive learning experiences such as simulations. Teachers can facilitate learning by providing learner support in the form of cueing (providing hints and a direction) during the simulation experience and conducting a guided reflection time following the simulation experience. Guided reflection is structured to provide feedback to students about their decision making but is also a time for learners to reflect on their experience, emotions, and clinical competency. Reflection time can vary, but because of its importance it should be given at least the same amount of time as the simulation itself (i.e., 20-minute simulation, 20-minute guided reflection).

Although the literature does not define the teacher's role very specifically in this context, it is known that the instructor is an integral part of any simulation. Weis and Guyton-Simmons (1998) during computer-based simulated experiences discussed how students solved problems better when a faculty member was present. Depending on whether the simulation is being conducted for learning or evaluation purposes, the teacher's role during the process will vary. However, unlike the traditional classroom, the instruction is no longer teacher-centered, but student-centered, with the teacher playing the role of a facilitator in the students' learning process. Teacher facilitation in distance learning can take place in numerous ways such as posting in discussion forums, through listservs, live chat rooms, or just simple e-mails sent to the individual students.

Educators must be prepared and feel comfortable with the simulations they are designing and implementing. Immersing educators into a simulation can allow the teachers to experience feelings similar to those of students, enabling them to understand students' anxiety and discomfort related to the simulation experience. To assume the role of the teacher in simulations, educators may require assistance in relation to design and activities, use of the technology, and setting up of the simulation and equipment.

The Learner's Role

Learners need to have specific information about the roles they are to play, particularly if the students are to work in groups. In simulations, learners usually play specific roles within the activity, with the roles varying from case to case. The literature suggests anywhere from 2 to 6 participants in a simulation. Learners can rotate through assigned roles in addition to talking about the various roles during the guided reflection time. Cioffi (2001) discussed two learner roles (response-based and process-based) when simulations are implemented in clinical practice. In the response-based role, the learner is not an active participant and has no control over the data presented. An example of this type of presentation would be assigning a student an observer role. These learners would not be active participants during the simulation, but could provide responses during the guided reflection on their perceptions of how the scenario unfolded. In the process-based method, the learners are active participants in the simulation, such as through patient role-plays or being assigned active roles in the simulated activities. In distance education settings, roles can be assigned for a particular debate, for example, an ethical, legal topic that is seen in nursing today. Students can be assigned roles to take part in this debate online and post accordingly in the discussion forum.

SIMULATION: A TEACHING-LEARNING INTERVENTION

As early as the late 1970s simulation was recognized as an effective training technique for critical skills such as those used in military maneuvers and flying. Over the last decade, simulation has been gaining acceptance as an invaluable educational tool for health care students because through the use of simulation students can be better prepared to provide competent and safe care for their patients.

In the late 1970s, when many of today's nursing educators were students in skills laboratories, few students probably thought of the mannequin in the nursing lab's hospital bed as anything but an occupant. Likewise, their instructors probably saw the same mannequin as simply a physical object to be turned and manipulated as students practiced the art of making an occupied bed. Not only has our conceptualization of the educational potential of simulation grown and matured in subsequent decades, but also the array of simulation modalities has multiplied. Partial-task trainers such as haptic IV start trainers and blood pressure arms assist students to achieve competence and confidence in the performance of a skill. Computer-assisted technology employs software that can challenge the user to apply knowledge and skills and to use critical thinking in real time (Seropian, 2003). Full-bodied computerized and interactive human patient simulators are now affordable and prevalent in nursing learning resource centers and provide a physiologically accurate and realistic representation of a human patient.

The importance of integrating simulation into nursing education is based on the fact that adequate clinical learning cannot be accomplished in the clinical arena alone (Carthew, 1998). Shortened hospital stays, increased patient loads, use of sophisticated technology on inpatient divisions, lack of appropriate professional nurse role models, and increased student enrollment all contribute to the problem of new graduates not being well prepared to handle the demands of the clinical care area. Using simulation as a teaching tool promotes the acquisition of skills that can better prepare the novice nurse. Students can be exposed to a baseline set of experiences, from fundamental core skills to complex scenarios, and evaluated in the mastery of fundamental as well as advanced challenges that require students to apply knowledge and utilize critical-thinking skills. The simulation activities ideally include working as a member of the health care team. The instructor provides feedback and redirects the student in the controlled environment. No harm can come to the patient. For these reasons, simulations are already being used for competency testing for health professionals (Issenberg et al., 1999).

The literature contains examples of simulation being used in the teaching-learning process for emergent care skills in health care programs, particularly in medical education. Gordon (2000) described a program at the University of Michigan where medical students were exposed to training scenarios designed to assist them to prepare for the care of acutely ill patients. In Melbourne, Australia, high-fidelity human patient simulation was used to help students learn to care for patients experiencing a medical crisis, such as hemorrhagic shock (Flanagan, Nestal, & Joseph, 2004). Other sources describe computer-assisted simulation employed to assist students to acquire and retain advanced cardiac life support (ACLS) skills (Schwid, Rooke, Ross, & Silvarajan, 1999).

In addition to preparing students for medical crises, simulation has been used as a strategy to prepare students for performing foundational skills and acquiring core knowledge. Carthew (1998) examined the role of the skills laboratory as a setting in which beginning students work on foundational skill attainment. She maintained that, with mastery of a full set of core psychomotor skills, students gain confidence and are more likely to perform efficiently in an actual patient care encounter. At Griffith University in Brisbane, Australia, clinical simulations are used to help beginning students develop problem-solving and clinical decision-making skills (Conrick, Dunne, & Skinner, 2004). Recognizing the enormous interest in using simulation and simulation products in nursing learning resource centers, some of which are very expensive, the National League for Nursing (NLN) and the Laerdal Corporation, an international leader in medical educational and total training products, together sponsored a national multisite, multimethod study to develop and test models using simulation to promote student learning in nursing (NLN, Laerdal, 2003). Other primary purposes of the project include developing a cadre of nursing faculty who can use simulations that enhance student learning; and contributing to the refinement of the body of knowledge related to the use of simulation in nursing education (NLN, Laerdal, 2003).

The skilled nursing professional must demonstrate competence across three domains: psychomotor, affective, and cognitive. Initially the use of simulation in clinical labs focused on the development of psychomotor skills to prepare beginning students for clinical experiences. However, the advantages of simulation have more frequently been reported in affective and cognitive domains. Although the literature to date contains few quantitative evaluations of simulation, anecdotal and subjective examples are easily found.

Affective Domain

Students who have experienced simulation instruction want more opportunities to learn in this manner (Conrick et al., 2004; Gordon, 2000). Students required to participate in a simulation report feeling performance anxiety yet appreciate that this learning experience provides more safety to their actual patients (Conrick et al., 2004). Consistently, students report greater confidence and self-efficacy in the protected environment (Mayne et al., 2004; Weiner, Gordon, & Gilman, 1993).

Cognitive Domain

Simulation as a teaching-learning intervention increases critical-thinking skills and sound clinical judgment (Bruce, Bridges, & Holcomb, 2003). Additionally, studies report better acquisition of knowledge in general (Weiner et al., 1993). The literature often compares simulation experiences as an aid to knowledge retention to traditional instructional experiences alone (Schwid et al., 1999). Working in complexly designed scenarios, students in one study appeared to demonstrate a sense of the value of professional teamwork and displayed an effort to provide holistic care (Mayne et al., 2004). Another study found that students studied more using simulation than they did with traditional textbook resources (Schwid et al., 1999).

Psychomotor Domain

From fundamental skill sets to complex and realistic scenarios, the use of simulation affords students the ability to practice in a protected and controlled environment as they progress through the nursing curriculum.

Students can be exposed to a full set of skills, including practicing emergent medical crises under the supervision and with the guidance of a faculty member in a "do no harm" environment. Motor skills and the use of highly technical equipment found in the acute and critical care settings can be practiced repeatedly without risk or inconvenience to patients through an assigned preceptor in their locations, yet the student can learn the content related to the skills through an online platform.

From the educator's perspective, except for the use of the most simple task trainer, the architecture of a simulation experience is an enormous challenge. However, evidence suggests that students are helped to bridge the theory-practice gap, retain information better, and show more self-confidence in beginning practice and desire to practice clinical skills. Faculty who are experienced with using simulation evaluate it as an efficacious and efficient method for measuring students' critical thinking and psychomotor skills. More research is needed to identify what components make up an ideal simulated environment, including the faculty role, and to quantify the learner outcomes when using simulation and how it is best used or blended with distance education. Faculty need technical and pedagogical support within schools of nursing in designing and implementing simulations for students at all levels.

SIMULATION: AN ENHANCEMENT
TO CLINICAL PRACTICE

Already noted were dynamics of the clinical area: increased staff workload, increased patient acuity, highly technical environment, shortened patient stays, and demands of increased nursing enrollments that limit the clinical facility's ability to be an ideal learning environment. Although research showing the effects of simulation on clinical performance is not well established, studies have shown positive effects on students' confidence as well as on student learning. A study of the impact of an interactive videodisc simulation on the confidence and knowledge of junior maternity students revealed the positive impact of the preparatory simulation preceding clinical experience over student clinical experience alone (Weiner et al., 1993). At Bell College of Health Studies in Dumfries, Australia, the challenge of greatly increased numbers of nursing students needing foundational experiences was met by providing a skills week (Mayne et al., 2004). In the context of case studies, the students made care decisions and practiced skills while learning about teamwork. A study by medical educators at the University of Texas at Galveston described the preparation of students in cardiopulmonary physical examination skills.

The educators, driven by the belief that "bedside teaching is becoming a lost art," turned to a simulation program for instruction, practice, and assessment (Karnath, Thorton, & Frye, 2002).

The international threat of terrorism has expanded nursing roles related to disaster nursing. Thankfully, this clinical training venue seldom exists and therefore simulation is employed to train health care professionals. Two programs—the Joint Trauma Training Center and United States Air Force Nursing Warskills Simulation Laboratory—use simulation as a teaching modality to ensure that nurses are prepared to respond to international medical disasters. Learning outcomes testing critical decision-making and trauma skills show that both programs are successful in preparing nurses to provide care to critically injured military personnel and civilians (Bruce et al., 2003).

The trend to enter advanced practice roles early in one's career means that the student does not bring a wealth of professional experience learned from years of practice to the graduate study setting. Simulation experiences representing situational realities of practice can be used effectively to develop skills previously learned from practice experience. Miller, Wilber, Dedhiya, Talashek, and Mrtek (2004) used simulated patients (SPs) to assess the interpersonal skills of nurse practitioner students. They found the experience to be profitable for these students, who benefited from the immediate and candid feedback offered by the SPs. In a distance education setting, the encounters with the SPs can be videotaped and linked to the content in order for the learner to assess the interpersonal skills of the caregivers in the vignette. The videotaped activity can also provide a mentoring model emphasizing good interpersonal skills for the learner.

In general, the factor that determines whether an individual has no skill, some skill, or complete mastery of a skill is the amount of deliberate practice that that person has completed (Issenberg et al., 1999). One problem in health care education has been that the situational practice usually involved a real patient. This problem creates the need for new methods of instruction, knowledge acquisition, and assessment of students. Advances in simulation technology as well as advances in pedagogical knowledge concerning how to use simulations present new tools and new methods for overcoming this challenge. Unlike patients, simulators do not become embarrassed, stressed, or injured; have predictable behavior; are available at any time to fit curriculum needs; can be programmed to simulate selected findings, conditions, situations, and complications; allow standardized experience for all trainees; can be used repeatedly with fidelity and reproducibility; and can be used to train individuals and teams for procedures and difficult management situations (Issenberg et al., 1999).

SIMULATION: AN ASSESSMENT METHOD

Simulations are increasingly being used in assessment of health profession-als (Schuwirth & van der Vleuten, 2003). Ever since the use of simulation in preparing health care professionals began in anesthesia, there is consid-erable information in the anesthesia literature about the use of simulation in performance assessment (Byrne & Greaves, 2001). The use of simula-tion in assessment falls into two broad categories: low-stakes and high-stakes situations (Boulet & Swanson, 2004). These assessments may use a range of simulation technologies, from case studies and standardized patients to haptic task trainers and high-fidelity human simulators. Low-stakes assessments are situations where the simulation is used by the learner or faculty to mark progress toward personal, course, or program learning goals. High-stakes assessments include licensing and certification examinations, credentialing processes, and employment decisions. As with any type of assessment, issues of validity and reliability must be considered (Boulet et al., 2003; Clauser, Kane, & Swanson, 2002).

For low-stakes assessments, construct and concurrent validity should be addressed. Construct validity is the degree to which an assessment instrument measures the dimensions of knowledge or skill development intended. Concurrent validity is determined by evaluating the relationship between how individuals perform on the new assessment (in this case a simulation) and the traditional (standard) assessment instrument. An example of how this concurrent validity can be evaluated is following a learning exercise, a pelvic exam for example, students would be asked to perform the exam on a simulator (e.g., METI's ExamSim) and on a standardized patient (Pugh & Youngblood, 2003). An assessment with high concurrent validity is one in which the learner's simulator assessment score is comparable to the score attained when performing the same exam on a standardized patient, using an accepted scoring checklist.

Predictive validity is required for simulations used in high-stakes assessments. Determining predictive validity is a complex process that takes a significant amount of time and can be quite expensive. Predictive validity is the extent to which performance on a particular simulation predicts a future performance, such as decision making or psychomotor skillfulness in a real-world clinical situation. Evaluating predictive validity requires that in addition to performance on the simulation, clinical skill or decision making of specific individuals be tracked over time. Assess-ment of the clinical performance over time is required so that a calculation can be made of the degree of certainty that one can have about the ability of the performance on a simulation to predict future performance.

Evaluating the reliability of assessments conducted using simulation can be difficult. In order to determine the reliability, or reproducibility, it is necessary to control all aspects of the simulation. A major aspect of this control is the degree of immersion created by the simulation. Immersion helps learners to suspend disbelief, or to forget that it is just a simulation, so that reproducible responses result.

SIMULATIONS: A BLENDED TEACHING-LEARNING MODEL WITH DISTANCE EDUCATION

The impact of the World Wide Web on nursing education has been significant. Many researchers (Chaffin & Maddux, 2004; Lindeman, 2000) believe this is an era of rapid change for nursing education, with the technology being the change agent. This shifting paradigm, teaching and learning via the Internet, coupled with the increased use of simulations and simulated learning, has great implications for nursing education.

Nursing education is no longer limited to the domain of the university, college, or hospital classroom. Education can be accessed in many cases through the Internet using asynchronous communication, e-mail, listservs, newsgroups, and conferencing (Carlton & Miller, 1999). Just a decade ago, there was much uncertainty with learning on the Internet; however, today nontraditional innovation in nursing is ever present. New modes of instructional methods using technology have arrived, such as the use of personal data assistants (PDAs) to retrieve and store information and resources (Thomas, Coppola, & Feldman, 2001); the use of the Internet for students to obtain a clinical practicum and instruction (Baier & Mueggenburg, 2001; Billings & Jeffries, 2004); health assessments being performed worldwide using the Internet (Scherubel, 2001); instruction on suturing wounds using virtual reality (Parvati et al., 2002); certification renewal in special procedures using simulators in an online environment (Thacker, 2004); and remediation for struggling students using the online environment and a patient simulator (Haskvitz & Koop, 2004).

Nursing educators value simulated teaching and learning. Clinical and community instruction have been a core part of educating nursing students for many years. Nurse educators have employed numerous interactive, experiential, simulated processes in the classroom such as role-play, using case scenarios (Lee & Lamp, 2003; Tomey, 2003), simulations reenacting realistic scenarios (Morton, 1999), gaming (Foster & Hardy, 1997), and other interactive activities. Nursing educators have also incorporated various modes of media and technology into the educational process such as PowerPoint presentations, videos, Webcasting, and the use of electronic portfolios. The interactive teaching-learning strategy in this section combines these two educational traditions—simulated learning with the technological. Selected examples of the blended use of simulated learning (e.g., use of simulations) and technological learning (i.e., use of distance education) will be described, as well as nursing implications of this educational strategy.

Background

Commercial CD-ROM programs designed to teach various skills and nursing concepts have emerged over the years. These products are typically two-dimensional, providing information to the learner in a convenient, accessible mode because the learner can review the content in class, at home, or in the learning laboratory. CD-ROMs are similar to videotapes; however, they include the capacity for learner interaction, producing active rather than passive learning.

More sophisticated products have been developed for nurse educators that include high-fidelity patient simulators. Nurse educators are now using patient simulators to provide students with practice experience in more realistic clinical settings. With the high-fidelity mannequins, the learner can hear heart and breath sounds, visualize an arrhythmia on a heart monitor, and palpate pulses. This experiential learning method is bringing more realism to the instruction and also elevating the learning experience to promote problem-solving and decision-making skills.

The Blended Approach

A new model of education arises when the two instructional strategies, use of technology and simulated learning, are wedded. No longer does the student have to be in a laboratory setting to practice assessment skills or drive many miles on a given day to achieve recertification of a skill or practice the technique of performing a 12-lead ECG or suturing an abdominal wound. Combining the Internet and the use of simulated learning offers great potential learning experiences to students of this generation.

At the University of California, Davis School of Medicine and Medical Center, students are getting the opportunity to practice invasive procedures that are complex skill-intensive via simulation (Thacker, 2004). Students currently perform the angioplasty and stent procedure on a patient simulator in a controlled lab setting; however, in the future they could perform the same procedure using a haptic device, with the program being accessed via the Internet.

Simulations accessed from a Web site are very important to nursing education today. For example, one Web site teaches the learner about 12-lead ECGs and how to interpret cardiac rhythms (Lindsey, 2004); another teaches learners about lung sounds (McGill University, n.d.). In the very recent past, clinical faculty would search high and low for a patient who had abnormal breath sounds, with only a few students then being able to gather around the patient for the learning experience. These Web sites with the simulated ECG and lung sounds now provide educators consistent, high-quality content for this type of instruction. In addition to these selected Web sites that demonstrate teaching via the computer and Internet, there are a variety of instructional strategies on the Web for students to access and use to enhance their knowledge.

There are also faculty-made CD-ROMS that can be used to supplement course materials. Wound assessment (Ross & Tuovinen, 2001), 12-lead ECGs (Jeffries et al., 2003), and cardiovascular aspects of nursing (Sternberg & Meyer, 2001) are available to provide experiential simulated learning to students. In Web courses, CD-ROMS are often provided to the learner to access the skill or a link is designed to connect the content to the learning of the material to provide more interactive learning experiences in the lesson.

Medical and nursing schools as well as major health care organizations are maintaining extensive Websites for learning, references, and assessment information (Parvati et al., 2002). Continuing medical and nursing education on the Internet is commonly available and a widely used service of practitioners. In one such case, the learning of anatomy and surgery is being taught for surgery interns via the Internet using a visuo-haptic-audio experience. Simulated environments are delivering the experience to the next generation of students in new innovative technological-enhanced learning environments.

Realistic simulations of tissue deformation and similar problems encountered in surgery are being delivered over a server with one gigabyte of memory and transmitted from the Internet to the user's workstation (Parvati et al., 2002). Interactive tools and collaborative software have been developed for this method of teaching and learning. Students can use a virtual tool (forceps) to pull on and distort a simulated model of an aorta within a model of an abdomen. The possibilities for manipulation and interaction within the program are phenomenal and promote a new, sophisticated type of teaching and learning.

The blend of technological advances and simulated learning is in the embryonic stage of delivery and use in the health care settings. For now, these innovative strategies are being used despite little evaluation data or evidence of optimal learning outcomes. However, just as with any innovation, the research will be conducted and outcomes will be studied and reported. In the meantime, as these technologies and strategies advance, educators need to be aware of the technology opportunities and ask how they may be used best in the nursing educational environment. Table 5.2 describes current nursing implications of the blended use of simulated and technological teaching and learning.

SUMMARY/CONCLUSIONS

A wide range of simulation technologies have become ubiquitous in the education and ongoing training of nurses and other health professionals. These technologies allow educators to develop effective and efficient strategies to teach decision making and clinical skills to diverse groups of students in complex simulated patient situations. Simulation is a strategy to engage students in active learning, which can be a significant challenge for students enrolled in programs of study that are "delivered"

TABLE 5.2   Nursing Implications of a Blended Education Model of Simulated and Technological Strategies

- Realize that as students gain more experience with technologies used in distance education, their expectations and experiences may change.
- Use formative, multidimensional strategies to evaluate the effects of new technologies and instructional strategies.
- Remember that students still have non-technology concerns about their learning—use evaluation components that address multiple components.
- Encourage programs and schools to develop comprehensive evaluation plans to gain information on complex interactions that occur with technological and simulated learning.
- Promote class discussion, which is critical for successful learning and allowing students to share knowledge, during their distance education work.
- Provide feedback, which is very important when interacting with students in a distance education model.
- Recognize roles may change periodically in the blended environment of technological and simulated learning: Students may become teachers and teachers become learners.
- Recognize opportunities to create online learning communities when blending simulated and technological learning, e.g., peer reviews, debates, resource sharing, etc.
- Ensure that faculty members undergo the simulated and technological learning experience created and assigned so they understand students' experience better.

at a distance. Initially, educators may resist use of simulation technologies because they may seem to create more work. Simulation does require one to consider the goals, the strategies needed to achieve the goals, and a method to evaluate whether or not goals were met.

Simulation as both a teaching-learning strategy and an approach to assessment has the advantage of actively engaging learners as individuals or as group members. Although usually thought of as an enhancement to clinical experience, simulation allows many clinical programs to be offered at a distance because it allows for a common, standardized way to assess all learners similarly, wherever they may be located. Although there has been an ever-increasing demand for distance education, hybrid or blended approaches to education developed and are responsive to consumers need for closeness and flexibility while permitting an objective way to assess experiential learning. Successful use of simulation, like successful distance education, requires a commitment on behalf of both the educators and the learners.

REFERENCES

Baier, M., & Mueggenburg, K. (2001). Using the Internet for clinical instruction. *Nurse Educator, 26*, 3.

Billings, D., & Jeffries, P. R. (2004). Learning marketspace partnerships: An Education Service Association model for developing online courses to prepare nurses for clinical practice in high demand specialties. Manuscript submitted for publication.

Billings, D., Jeffries, P. R., Daniels, D., Reising, D., Stanley, T., Stone, C., & Stephenson, E. (in press, 2005). Developing and using online courses to prepare nurses for employment in critical care. *Journal of Staff Development Nursing.*

Boulet, J. R., Murray, D., Kras, J., Woodhouse, J., McAllister, J., & Ziv, A. (2003). Reliability and validity of a simulation-based acute care skills assessment for medical students and residents. *Anesthesiology, 99*, 1270–1280.

Boulet, J. R., & Swanson, D. B. (2004). Psychometric challenges of using simulations in high-stakes assessment. In W. F. Dunn (Ed.), *Simulation in critical care and beyond* (pp. 119–130). Des Plains, IL: Society of Critical Care Medicine.

Bruce, S., Bridges, E., & Holcomb, J. B. (2003). Preparing to respond: Joint trauma training center and USAF nursing warskills simulation laboratory. *Critical Care Nursing Clinics of North America, 15*, 149–162.

Byrne, A. J., & Greaves, J. D. (2001). Assessment instruments used during anaesthetic simulation: Review of published studies. *British Journal of Anaesthesiology, 86*, 445–450.

Carlton, K., & Miller, P. A. (1999). Connecting points: Asynchronous communication. *Computers in Nursing, 17*, 162–165.

Carthew, L. (1998). The clinical practice suite and clinical skills: Preparation for pre-registration students of nursing. Retrieved November 10, 2004, from ww.hpw.org.uk/images_client/Lillian_Carthew.pdf

Chaffin, A. J., & Maddux, C. D. (2004). Internet teaching methods for use in baccalaureate nursing education. *Computers in Nursing, 22,* 132–144.

Cioffi, J. (2001). Clinical simulations: Development and validation. *Nurse Education Today, 21,* 477–486.

Clauser, B., Kane, M., & Swanson, D. (2002). Validity issues for performance-based tests scored with computer-automated scoring systems. *Applied Measurement in Education, 15,* 413–432.

Conrick, M., Dunne, A., & Skinner, J. (2004). Learning together: Using simulation to foster integration of theory and practice. *Australian Electronic Journal of Nursing Education, 1*(1).

Engum, S., & Jeffries, P. R. (2003). Intravenous catheter training system: Computer-based education vs. traditional learning methods. *American Journal of Surgery, 186*(1), 67–74.

Flanagan, B., Nestal, D., & Joseph, M. (2004). Making patient safety the focus: Crisis resource management in the undergraduate curriculum. *Medical Education, 38*(1), 56–66.

Foster, H., & Hardy, N. (1997). Crisis simulation and health care systems, *Simulations and Gaming, 28*(2), 198–199.

Gordon, J. A. (2000). The human patient simulator: Acceptance and efficacy as a teaching tool for students. *Academic Medicine, 75,* 522.

Haskvitz, L., & Koop, E. (2004). Students struggling in clinical? A new role for the patient simulator. *Journal of Nursing Education, 43,* 181–184.

Hovancsek, M., Horn, M., Jamison, R., & Narsavage, G. (2004). *A comparison of two simulation methods for teaching intravenous cannulation.* Poster session presented at the Biennial North American Learning Resource Conference, Spokane, WA.

Issenberg, B. S., McGaghie, W. C., Hart, I. R., Mayer, J. W., Felner, J. M., Petrusa, E. R., et al. (1999). Simulation technology for health care professional skills training and assessment. *Journal of the American Medical Association, 282,* 861–866.

Jeffries, P., Woolf, P., & Linde, B. (2003). Technology-based vs. traditional instruction: A comparison of two methods for teaching the skill of performing a 12-lead ECG. *Nursing Education Perspective, 24*(2), 70–74.

Karnath, B., Thorton, W., & Frye, A. (2002). Teaching and testing physical examination skills without the use of patients. *Academic Medicine, 77,* 753.

Lee, C., & Lamp, J. (2003). The use of humor and role-playing in reinforcing key concepts. *Nurse Educator, 28*(2), 61.

Lindeman, C. A. (2000). The future of nursing education. *Journal of Nursing Education, 39,* 5–12.

Lindsey, A. (2004). *ECG learning center in cyberspace.* Retrieved December 12, 2004, from http://medstat.med.utah.edu/kw/ecg/ecg_outline/

Mayne, W., Jooton, D., Young, B., Harland, G., Harris, M., & Lyttle, C. (2004). Enabling students to develop confidence in basic clinical skills. *Nursing Times, 100*(24), 36–39.

McGill University Virtual Stethoscope. Retrieved December 10, 2004, from http://nursing.about.com/gi/dynamic/offsite.htm?site=http%3A%2F%2Fsprojects.mmi.mcgill.ca%2Fmvs%2Fmvsteth.htm

Miller, A. M., Wilber, J., Dedhiya, S., Talashek, M. L., & Mrtek, R. (2004). Interpersonal styles of nurse practitioner students during simulated patient encounters. *Clinical Excellence for Nurse Practitioners, 2*, 166–171.

Morton, P. (1999). Using a critical care simulation laboratory to teach students, *Critical Care Nurse, 17*(6), 66–68.

National League for Nursing and Laerdal Corporation. (2003). Designing and implementing models for the innovative use of simulation to teach nursing care of ill adults and children: A national multi-site, multi-method study. Six Month Progress Report. Reporting Period, June 1, 2003 to December 31, 2003.

Parvati, D., Montgomery, K., Senger, S., Heinrichs, W., Srivastava, S., & Waldron, K. (2002). Simulated medical learning environments on the Internet. *Journal of the American Medical Informatics Association, 9*, 437–447.

Pugh, C. M., & Youngblood, P. (2003). Development and validation of assessment measures for a newly developed physical examination simulator. *Journal of the American Medical Informatics Association, 9*, 448–460.

Ross, G. C., & Tuovinen, J. E. (2001). Deep versus surface learning with multimedia in nursing education: Development and evaluation of wound care. *Computers in Nursing, 19*, 213–223.

Scherubel, J. C. (2001). A global health analysis project for baccalaureate nursing students. *Journal of Professional Nursing, 17*, 96–100.

Schuwirth, L. W., & van der Vleuten, C. P. (2003). The use of clinical simulations in assessment. *Medical Education, 37*(Suppl. 1), S65–S71.

Schwid, H. A., Rooke, G. A., Ross, B. K., & Silvarajan, M. (1999). Use of a computerized advanced cardiac life support simulation improves retention of advanced life support guidelines better than a textbook review. *Critical Care Medicine, 27*, 821–824.

Seropian, M. (2003). General concepts in full scale simulation: Getting started. *Anesthesiology Analog, 97*, 1695–1705.

Sternberg, C., & Meyer, L. (2001). Hypermedia-assisted instruction: Authoring with learning guidelines. *Computers in Nursing, 19*, 69–74.

Thacker, P. (2004). Fake worlds offer real medicine: Virtual reality finding a role in treatment and training. *Journal of the American Medical Association, 290*, 2107–2112.

Thomas, B. A., Coppola, J. F., & Feldman, H. (2001). Adopting handheld computers for community based curriculum: Case study. *Journal of New York State Nurses Association, 32*, 4–6.

Tomey, A. M. (2003). Learning with cases. *Journal of Continuing Education in Nursing, 34*(1), 34–38.

Wakefield, A., Cooke, S., & Biggs, C. (2003). Learning together: Use of simulated patients with nursing and medical students for breaking bad news. *International Journal of Palliative Nursing, 9*(1), 22–28.

Weiner, E., Gordon, J., & Gilman, D. (1993). Evaluation of a labor and delivery videodisc simulation. *Computers in Nursing, 11*, 191–196.

Weis, P., & Guyton-Simmons, J. (1998). A computer simulation for teaching critical thinking skills. *Nurse Educator, 23*(2), 30–33.

CHAPTER 6

Using Learning Objects to Enhance Distance Education

Tami H. Wyatt and Linda Royer

A student whom we will call Mark is struggling with the concept of levels of prevention in health care. He visits the course Web site and clicks on a "jewel" in an overflowing treasure chest marked LOP (levels of prevention). The screen opens to the scene of a climber scaling a mountain, which has plateaus at various points in the climb. In the foothills, the first plateau is called Primary Prevention Overlook. When the mouse is moved over the signpost, a drop-down menu gives a definition. Moving the mouse over the adjacent telescopic viewer opens a box that provides operational examples relating to the mountain-climbing experience but parenthetically contrasting with maintaining health. Further into the climb, the next plateau reveals a similar pattern but with reference to increasing risk and consequences on the Secondary Prevention Overlook. And at the peak, the Tertiary Prevention Overlook describes more increasing challenges and consequences to individuals and society.

Mark has just experienced a learning object in the quest for knowledge. It has satisfied his need for visual stimulus and has challenged his critical thinking in comprehending increasingly complex concepts. And it has taken 5 minutes of his time. It will be there for Susan, Joy, Allen, and others. It is an elaborate example of pedagogy that is especially appealing to a profession experiencing diminishing resources—nursing education.

So what is a learning object? A simple Internet search for the term "learning objects" (LOs), or "reusable learning objects" (RLOs), quickly reveals that the concept has emerged among educators in the last 6 years and is fiercely debated. The logical starting point in understanding a learning object is to define it. This would appear to be a fairly simple task, yet it is not, because the definition of a learning object is precisely where the debate begins, depending on the philosophical structure of various educational communities. Because of and despite the debates surrounding LOs, an exploration of learning objects is worthwhile because they are being used extensively in higher education. Furthermore, nursing education is rapidly expanding into distance education and resources that enhance this modality should be examined, including lessons learned from other disciplines.

There are challenges in teaching faculty to adopt ever more sophisticated technology into the curriculum, such as how to (a) recognize learning needs to utilize technology in the context of the intended theory or content, (b) bring clarity and purpose in the use of technology aids, (c) apply the knowledge in increasingly sophisticated methods through advancing levels of cognition, and (d) divide learning information into "chunks." Adult learners bring varying cognitive abilities (learning styles), demands for convenience and expediency, time constraints, expectations for immediacy, and various levels of education skills. Learners have a broad range of creativity, writing, and critical thinking skills; time management and study habit deficits; and a range of motivation to achieve. Educators are recognizing that methods are needed to help learners retain 80% of knowledge that is forgotten over time.

The purpose of this chapter is to stimulate interest in a new method of content development though technology, namely, learning objects. The objectives are to define and explain LOs and their standards; why learning objects are suitable for nursing curricula; suggest how faculty communities may adopt their usage; and provide Internet resources for using, creating, and storing LOs.

DEFINING LEARNING OBJECTS

A learning object is a small unit of content with its description of usability or application employed for teaching and learning. It has been described as analogous to Legos building blocks in which a variety of shapes may be creatively assembled by the visionary to form a creative object. In the case of education, the creator is the course content builder and the Lego pieces are the units, or building blocks, of knowledge. A learning object can be reused, altered for other purposes, and enhanced for sophistication—hence the name "reusable learning object"—and organized with other material or objects associated with learning objectives. Because this chapter deals with the use of learning objects in distance education, the definition should include any digital object (audio, video, image, text, or any combination) that enhances learning and meets an objective. A learning object that is computer-based can be used by multiple learners and educators and revisions can be accessed immediately (Wiley, 2000). Bear in mind that an LO is raw data and requires a system to organize it. It is not a medium to deliver instruction like a digital slide presentation is (PowerPoint, for instance) or a course management system (i.e., WebCT, Blackboard, etc.). Rather, a learning object is one of the several methods an educator will use to explain an objective. Because of its digital design, it enhances learning and may be delivered synchronously or asynchronously through a course management system (CMS) also known as learning management system (LMS) or learning content management system (LCMS). It is worth mentioning a few of the most frequently cited definitions in order to gain a clearer understanding of the differences and complexities surrounding learning objects.

The International Electrical and Electronic Engineering Association (IEEE) offers one of the most widely quoted definitions: a learning object is any entity, digital or nondigital, which can be used, reused, or referenced during technology-supported learning. Although this definition is widely accepted, it is broad and illuminates little of what a learning object is or what it is not.

David Wiley, an expert on learning objects, provides a more general definition: a learning object is any digital resource that can be reused to support learning (Wiley, 2000). But it is more than that: a description of the way in which it is used must accompany it to make it reusable. And the author of learning objects, Wayne Hodgins of Worldwide Learning Strategies, challenges educators to apply a high level of "creatability" in their development that may be applicable to the unexpected in the world of knowledge sharing. He speaks of availability everywhere, every time, to everyone—an Any-to-Every concept.

Although definitions vary, most authorities on learning objects describe three principles that should be present in all learning objects (Polsani, 2003):

1. interoperability—the ability to effectively and efficiently use content from multiple sources within different systems (Eduworks, 2004).

2. reusability—the ability to use a learning object in multiple contexts

3. accessibility—the ability to access learning objects easily through stored and referenced databases

These principles are necessary for the adoption of learning objects, which when properly used and shared are cost-effective, time efficient, and promote effective teaching and learning (Christiansen & Anderson, 2004).

STANDARDS FOR LEARNING OBJECTS

An influential group comprised of the Learning Technology Standards Committee of IEEE, IMS Global Learning Consortium, and the Dublin Core Metadata Initiative has developed metadata standards for learning object creation, storage, and retrieval (Polsani, 2003). Metadata standards refer to the guidelines for creating data about data. More simply stated, metadata files are text-rich files that provide a universal nomenclature for organizing learning objects. Without standards for metadata files and learning objects, they cannot be adopted by multiple users, in multiple contexts, and in multiple arenas.

The Sharable Content Object Reference Model (SCORM) is a set of guidelines with specifications and standards that encourage a common technical framework for computer and Web-based learning. Specifically, SCORM describes a content aggregation model (CAM) and run-time environment (RTE) for learning objects to be adaptable in multiple ways (Advanced Distributive Learning, 2003). SCORM meets universal standards for metadata so that databases or repositories that house learning objects may be harvested and converted to other storage repositories easily.

Beyond the metadata and learning objects standards described above, more specific standards with a controlled naming scheme must be created by the learning objects developers. These specific guidelines are typically discipline-specific and use nomenclature similar to that of electronic library databases such as MEsH headings used in Medline. This ensures a universal naming and organizing system so that various databases and repositories of learning objects can be shared among institutions and educators.

LEARNING OBJECTS IN NURSING EDUCATION

Learning objects are well suited for nursing education, especially those curricula exploring distance education. For nursing programs to gain recognition through accrediting bodies and to meet standards set forth by the National Board of Nursing, educational programs must vary minimally from one program to the next. In fact, programs must comply with specific curriculum content. Conceptual models of nursing and nursing theory and ethical principles are drawn upon at increasing level of sophistication in the education experience. Based on these facts, the sharing and reusing of teaching/learning concepts is not only feasible but sound practice for cost-effectiveness and resource allocation. Thorough and meticulous planning is essential before adopting learning objects so that the objects can be used, retrieved, and stored, and to ensure quality in the educational experience. This planning must consider not only learning objects but also the ways to organize and tag the objects (metadata), the ways learning objects are integrated in LCMSs, and it must occur in two domains: curriculum planning, and the planning of the creation, storage, and retrieval of learning objects.

Planning a Learning-Object-Rich Curriculum

As schools of nursing move further into the world of technological advances, reliance on digitally prepared teaching illustrations and tools gain acceptance and credibility for their cost-effective application. Educators who work with instructional designers and technology experts on campus are more likely to develop competence in the design, use, and reuse of learning objects. There must be a commitment to integrate the technology infrastructure of the institution and a vision of the creative potential inherent in this method of teaching to reap the benefits over the long term.

Ornstein and Hunkins (1998, pp. 204–205) describe several curriculum building models (for example, Bobbit, Charters, Tyler, Taba, Glatthorn) that readers may consider. For the purpose of this discussion, the authors will describe Glatthorn's naturalistic model, which has eight steps: (1) Assess the alternatives to what is currently used; (2) stake out the territory by defining the course parameters and the learning audience; (3) develop a collaborative constituency for the process that is inclusive and fosters growth; (4) build the knowledge base about the content, the students, faculty skill, participation by the technology department, and potential research opportunity; (5) block the units, courses, or modules of study for learner-based need; (6) plan quality learning experiences to address the objectives through student-centered approaches, allowing for flexibility according to learner needs; (7) develop the course assessments with student participation requirements such as portfolios, biographies, etc.; (8) develop the learning scenarios rather than the standard curriculum guide, such as learning contracts or learning plans.

The first domain of planning requires an evaluation of the program and specific needs to ensure the learning objects have contextual meaning and will transition smoothly into the curricula. The curriculum committee examines the philosophical underpinnings of the program, keeping in mind the constructivist approach and which digital-based learning components embody the requirements of adult learners and complement the curriculum. After careful consideration, the committee plans the systematic identification of existing raw data in the curriculum content. Faculty submit their wealth of illustrations, interactive methods, and learning assessment tools to share with the committee. The learning objects are evaluated for relevance and reuse or replicability in the progression of learning objectives. Collaborative work with technology experts in digital design and development of computer-based course management is essential in the second domain, which is the planning of the creation, storage, and retrieval of learning objects.

Planning the Creation, Storage, and Retrieval of Learning Objects

The second domain requires an examination of the program learning concepts so that the learning objects are interoperable, reusable, and accessible. Before creating learning objects, the associated objective must be broken into its smallest element (granularity), matching a learning object to a single learning entity or concept. Likewise, the learning object represents the smallest element of a learning resource. Wiley (2002) noted an inverse relationship between granularity or the size of the learning object and its reusability; the larger the learning object, the less the object is reused. Granularity of a learning object ensures effective utilization of the resources because objects are created at the smallest level of learning structure and can be used in a variety of ways to meet multiple learning objectives. LOs stored in repositories (libraries) of learning objects are easily accessible and cost-effective.

The director of an institution's resource center/medial laboratory plays a valuable role in creating a repository. Educators and technology experts view this method as cost-saving because the institution can do the following: "(1) develop and deploy learning content quickly and efficiently, (2) port content easily between multiple LMSs or LCMSs, (3) reduce content development and delivery costs, (4) reduce maintenance time and costs" (Mortimer, 2002).

There are a variety of methods to use in the creation of learning objects. Examples are given in Table 6.1, all dependent on the skill sets of faculty and technology experts. It may be as simple as a photo in a

TABLE 6.1   Scope of Learning Objects in Context of Bloom Taxonomy

Type	Measurable Behavior	Description	Required thinking level
Photo/clipart (scenario, face, symbol) Diagram, poster, illustration, outline	Recognize, describe, identify, locate, select, label, memorize, infer	Digital photo or graphic alone or imbedded in a presentation; can be manipulated for effect Conveying a concept or procedure of learning	Comprehension
Cartoon, animated story or procedure, snippet of movie, video	Add: Summarize, restate, paraphrase, match, explain, defend, compare, contrast, generalize Based on previous knowledge, may examine, classify, categorize, differentiate	Digital cartoon can be created in Flash™ or brief movie or video may be imbedded in PPT or presented in a viewer on Web page	Comprehension Analysis
Poll procedure, survey, interactive object manipulation	Compare, put together, disassemble, change, construct, sketch, solve, show, collect, prepare	In interactive polling or survey procedure where data are crunched with a background db engine; digital whiteboard online activities between teacher and learners; little Flash™ movie with viewer-manipulated objects	Application
Hyperlinks to Internet referencing or data mining	Question, examine, classify, categorize, research, differentiate, investigate	A report-building instruction set; a definition-building or critical thinking exercise	Analysis

(continued)

TABLE 6.1 *(continued)*

Type	Measurable Behavior	Description	Required thinking level
Interactive games, quizzes, tests, group projects online, simulation	Experiment, speculate, create, invent, combine Construct, originate, design, formulate, role-play, develop, propose	Can be created with Java script as pop-up boxes on a Web page or as a self-grading assessment in an LMS; groups may meet in discussion forums (asynchronous) or chat rooms (synchronous) environments	Synthesis
Posting of student reflections on learning experience, performance evaluations, debates, group discussions	Compare, recommend, assess, value, apprise, solve, criticize, weigh, consider, debate	Modalities may be discussion forums or chat, electronic survey, audio/video conferencing or reporting, electronic voting/polling	Evaluation

slide presentation or more technical such as a brief Flash movie embedded in a Web page or in a slide presentation. Once these assets are created, they should be treated as jewels in a treasure chest of resources. For that to occur, they need to be identified in relationship to (1) their use on all possible levels and (2) in all potential applications to knowledge-building related to the learning objectives; as well as (3) assessment of learning strategies, (4) file size or "seat time"—the time it takes to teach or the student to complete; and (5) its relationship to associated learning objects and the larger learning asset. The learning object should be established in a file structure similar to a library and supported with keywords and phrases that allow any faculty member to search for an illustration that enhances their teaching presentation. Quality learning objects that are effectively organized in a searchable repository contribute to the goal of just-in-time learning and many-to-every delivery.

Learning objects are easily stored on servers with Internet access. If material is copyright protected, databases or repositories that store the learning objects must be secure and require authentication with login pages. This protects the copyright and educational fair use practices. If learning objects are not copyright material, then open source repositories should be considered so that the learning objects are public domain, encouraging a community of sharing among nursing educators. The authors would go a step further and invite all schools of nursing to form consortiums for the purposes of sharing the wealth of learning objects extant and collaborate on effective and efficient development of new ones. Many hours of time and creative energy may be saved for the demand of student interaction in a resource-constrained profession.

All faculty and instructors may contribute to the development of learning objects, at any level of technological expertise. The learners themselves will have valid ideas for their design as well. Just as with the adoption of the distance learning modality into curricula, the acceptance of change in the delivery mode for personalized knowledge tools comes at a varying pace. A successful transition to the adoption of learning objects is aided by mentoring and sharing of creative ideas and expertise.

Once the scope of the best course resources, or course assets, are viewed and all possible applications of the tools of learning are matched to the curriculum threads, the process should be documented. Then the assets are broken down into data bits, or finer granularity. As discussed previously, all information about the data bit (LO) is documented using a table with suggested headings: title, description, author, date of creation, keywords/phrases or wordsense, related learning objective, where used (PPT, video, assessment, Web page, etc.), type of LO, language, estimated learning time. Once faculty have a clear view of existing assets of learning and their related LOs, creation may begin on additional LOs that further enhance the learning experiences of students. Admittedly, the early phase of curriculum revision as it relates to this computer technology demands effort and time and requires attention to the learning curve of faculty. Once procedures, resources, and scheduling are put in place, conceptualization, creation, and integration of new learning objects and their relativity to the curriculum become commonplace. The importance of creating a sharing culture through consortiums and working relationships with nurse educators across communities cannot be overemphasized. Without a sharing culture, resources are re-created again and again and resources are underutilized once created.

INTERNET RESOURCES FOR LEARNING OBJECTS

The authors wish to direct the readers to various resources on the Internet pertaining to learning objects. This list is not conclusive and by no means should be considered the only resources available. In fact, this simply scratches the surface of information on learning objects. However, the authors believe that this list provides a foundation for educators desiring more information about learning objects.

Tutorials and Presentations

AliveTek, Inc., Learning about Learning Objects through Learning Objects
http://www.alivetek.com/learningobjects.htm

Wisc-Online: Wisconsin Online Resource Center
http://www.wisc-online.com/index.htm

TechLearn 2001
http://www.eduworks.com/LOTT/tutorial/

University of Wisconsin-Center for International Education
http://www.uwm.edu/Dept/CIE/AOP/learningobjects.html

The University of Nottingham, School of Nursing Educational Technology Group
http://www.nottingham.ac.uk/nursing/sonet/rlos/

eLearning Curve Newsletter
http://www.icaxon.com/elearning/elnovember2001.html

Macromedia Learning Object Development Center
http://www.macromedia.com/resources/elearning/objects/

Technology for eLearning
http://ferl.becta.org.uk/display.cfm?page=307

Learning Standards Acronyms
http://www.learnativity.com/acronyms.html

Learning Objects Libraries/Repositories

Merlot: Multimedia Educational Resource for Learning and Online Teaching
http://www.merlot.org/artifact/BrowseArtifacts.po?firsttime=true

Health on the Net Foundation
http://www.hon.ch/HONmedia/

CAREO: Campus Alberta Repository of Educational Objects
http://careo.ucalgary.ca/cgi-bin/WebObjects/CAREO.woa

University of Wisconsin Institute for Global Studies
http://www.uw-igs.org/search/index.asp

University of Texas at San Antonio: List of Learning Objects
Repository
http://elearning.utsa.edu/guides/LO-repositories.htm

Interactive Health Tutorials
http://www.nlm.nih.gov/medlineplus/tutorial.html

University of Alberta, Learning Objects Repository
http://www.nursing.ualberta.ca/homepage.nsf/site?OpenView&
RestrictToCategory=Learning+Objects+Repository

Online LO Articles

The Instructional Use of Learning Objects
http://www.reusability.org/read/

Use and Abuse of Reusable Learning Objects
http://elearning.utsa.edu/guides/LO-repositories.htm

Designing Courses
http://www.ibritt.com/resources/dc_objects.htm

Beyond Institutional Boundaries: reusable learning objects for multi-
professional education
http://www.ucel.ac.uk/documents/docs/dublin_paper.pdf

EduSource: Canada's Learning Object Repository Network
http://www.itdl.org/Journal/Mar_04/article01.htm

A Field Guide to Learning Objects
http://www.learningcircuits.org/NR/rdonlyres/17DB7DB7-0E67-
480F-BA5C-4D0A2336529D/1091/smartforce.pdf

Preparing Teachers to Use Learning Objects
http://ts.mivu.org/default.asp?show=article&id=961

REFERENCES

Advanced Distributive Learning. (2003). *SCORM overview*. Retrieved September
27, 2004, from http://www.adlnet.org/index.cfm?fuseaction=scormabt

Christiansen, J. A., & Anderson, T. (2004, March). Feasibility of course development based on learning objects: Research analysis of three case studies. *International Journal of Instructional Technology and Distance Learning*, 04, Article
02. Retrieved from http://www.itdl.org/Journal/Mar_04/article02.htm

EduWorks. (2004). *All about learning objects: Online learning content*. Retrieved
September 17, 2004, from http://www.eduworks.com/LOTT/utorial/learning
objects.html

Mortimer, L. (2002). *(Learning) objects of desire: Promise and practicality.* Learning Circuits: American Society for Training and Development. Retrieved October 15, 2004, from http://www.learningcircuits.org/2002/apr2002/mortimer.html

Ornstein, A. C., & Hunkins, F. P. (1998). *Curriculum: Foundations, principles, and issues* (3rd ed.). Boston: Allyn and Bacon.

PGL Database Workshop: eLearning Objects and Systems, held by The Partnership in Global Learning in Orlando Florida June, 2004.

Polsani, P. R. (2003, February 19). Use and abuse of reusable learning objects. *Journal of Digital Information, 3*(4), article No. 164. Retrieved from http://jodi.ecs.soton.ac.uk/Articles/v03/i04/Polsani/

Wiley, D. A. (2000). Connecting learning objects to instructional design theory: A definition, a metaphor, and a taxonomy. In D. A. Wiley (Ed.), *The Instructional Use of Learning Objects* [Electronic version]. Retrieved September 17, 2004, from http://reusability.org/read/chapters/wiley.doc

Wiley, D. A. (2002). *The instructional use of learning objects.* Bloomington, IN: Agency for Instructional Technology and Association for Educational Communication & Technology.

CHAPTER 7

Motivation and Distance Education Students

Christine A. Hudak

NURSING AND DISTANCE EDUCATION

Proliferating Programs

Distance education courses in continuing nursing education programs are rapidly increasing in number and size. Universities traditionally devoted to on-campus education activities are joining the ranks of their nontraditional counterparts in offering associate, baccalaureate, master's, and doctoral programs fully or partially online. Additionally, the high cost and time constraints of hospitals in providing mandatory continuing education for nursing staff has spawned the development of companies providing online courses to meet all or a portion of a nurse's biennial education requirements for relicensure.

AACN's Position

The American Association of Colleges of Nursing (AACN) recognized the necessity of using distance education in today's varied education environments for nursing. In January 2000, the AACN published a bulletin entitled *Distance Education Is Changing and Challenging Nursing Education*. In it, the AACN cited multiple reasons for embracing the concept of distance education for entry, advanced, and continuing nursing education. Distance education is seen as remedy to the nursing shortage, an asset in the battle against shrinking nursing faculty numbers, a way to keep nurses working while pursuing advanced education, and a way of plugging the brain drain in many communities as their skilled workers and students leave for education and never return (AACN, 2000a). In the accompanying white paper, *Distance Technology in Nursing Education* (AACN, 2000b), the AACN defines distance education and distance education technologies and offers multiple factors for policy makers, external funders, educators in nursing and related fields, and health care institutions to consider. These varying supports for distance education by nursing educators, health care institutions, and nursing professionals themselves have been further enhanced by advances in technology.

Technological Enhancers

New and improved technologies such as digital subscriber lines (DSL) and cable modems have improved the speed and quality of Internet access. Web portals and virtual private networks (VPN) have made it possible to utilize applications such as WebCT or Blackboard to deliver real-time lectures, hold office hours, or engage in discussions in the synchronous mode. These same activities can be stored by these applications and utilized by learners unavailable in real time. This asynchronous mode allows distance learners to benefit from their classmates despite being unavailable during the real-time activities. Online lectures can be easily burned to a CD-ROM using Microsoft Publisher and then uploaded to a network or distributed to students in person or by mail. Desktop videoconferencing from a home or office computer makes individual or preceptor conferences as effortless as a phone call. Wireless networks allow students access to university libraries, Web portals, and instructional programs from multiple venues including neighborhood public libraries and the closest Starbucks. Cost decreases and the greater availability of technology make access to distance education a possibility and a reality for all who are motivated to participate. But what does motivate the learner to participate? Are the factors for distance education similar to those for traditional education, or are there characteristics of distance learners that make them different from the traditional learner? Before answering these questions, let us turn to a general discussion of student motivation for learning. Some answers may be found in previous educational research in adult education.

THE MIND-MOTIVATION CONNECTION: EXTRINSIC VERSUS INTRINSIC MOTIVATION

What motivates the learner? Perhaps the best place to start is with the physiologic basis for motivation. In *The Art of Changing the Brain* (Zull, 2002), this physiologic basis for motivation begins with the differentiation between extrinsic and intrinsic motivation. Although these concepts are not new to nursing educators, viewing them in a physiologic context provides a new dimension of knowledge.

Deception and Loss of Control

Extrinsic motivators can induce or persuade students to complete tasks that lead to learning. Intrinsic motivators are automatically connected to learning; we have evolved to want them (Zull, 2002). To illustrate this in light of the learner's brain, Zull offers the explanation about what happens when a student is offered a reward or punishment (an extrinsic motivator). The first thing seen by the brain of the student in this reward or punishment situation is a loss of control. This is not a conscious recognition, but one that the brain recognizes and attempts to suppress. It deciphers "deceptions like extrinsic rewards" (Zull, 2002, p. 53), and knows there is a substitution of an external reward for the actual internal decision to do something by the student, that is, learn. There is no longer any reason for the student to do the thing we have asked except to obtain the reward or avoid the punishment. To the student's brain, the offer of an extrinsic reward is a deception.

> The brain sees through the extrinsic reward. It sees the extrincity. The reward is tempting, true enough, so we devise all sorts of ways to get the reward without carrying out the education, the job, or the assignment. Students seem to do this quite effectively in our colleges. Sometimes they even get A's (the reward) in courses they hardly remember taking a few months later. (Zull, 2002, p. 53)

This is not to say that extrinsic rewards do not have their place, but because they are aimed at things outside learning (Zull, 2002), the use of these rewards should be creative and considered. As a first step in moving to intrinsic motivation for the student, extrinsic motivators can be quite useful.

Extrinsic to Intrinsic

As an example, a learner is considering whether or not to take a distance education class. This will involve changes in lifestyle, loss of free time, an output of a considerable sum of money, and probably most important, disruption of the status quo of the learner's current comfort zone. Though the loss of all these things can be disturbing, the learner may view as a payoff an extrinsic reward such as an increase in pay or a promotion. Rarely will the learner consider knowledge of a particular subject valuable for its own sake, and rarely will the pursuit of knowledge in a specific area lead to satisfaction. But if the learner strives to achieve the external reward (the extrinsic motivation), that same learner may find the actual pursuit of knowledge stimulating and enjoyable. Thus, an extrinsic motivator may serve as a bridge to the intrinsic motivator of enjoyment of a subject; a previously unengaged student may become engaged, enthusiastic, and excited about education.

That same learner, when faced with a particularly daunting education task, may also use extrinsic motivators to continue the task (Zull, 2002). Writing a research paper on an unknown topic may prove tedious and boring; studying pharmacology and epistemology may prove frustrating. However, the thought of an extrinsic reward, such as praise from the instructor or a high score on a pharmacology exam, may be the boost needed to keep the student pursuing the subject. Zull calls this "sustain[ing] a learner at times of pressure and difficulty" (2002, p. 53).

Motivation and the Distance Learner

Zull's premise about the connection between intrinsic rewards and education leads to a natural conclusion that if we want to help students learn, then we should find out what is already motivating them (Zull, 2002). If we don't and continue to offer only extrinsic rewards, then we take the chance of actually decreasing learning (Kohn, 1993). Following this traditional line of reasoning and applying it to distance education allows us to conclude that motivation for distance learners should be tied to something that already motivates them. The answer to this motivation question becomes the answer to the more basic question, Why do learners take distance education courses? Looking at the characteristics of distance learners provides more evidence.

DISTANCE LEARNER CHARACTERISTICS

Distance education is not a new concept; indeed, correspondence courses have been around for decades. Research on the characteristics of distance learners has also been conducted for decades. Unfortunately, this research has been sporadic and focused on concerns of individual universities and stakeholder groups rather than systematic or evaluative in nature (Roberts, Irani, Lundy, & Telg, 2003). What we are looking at in the field of distance education research is a multiplicity of studies with various learners and educational programs. We must be able to extract information from these studies that will be of use to distance education practitioners.

Until recently, most distance learners were considered mature and were identified by common characteristics such as valuing education and having high motivation, realistic expectations about the education experience, competing life interests, ingrained education patterns, life experience and a developed value system, and independence; and being achievement oriented and active learners (Benshoff & Lewis, 1992; Cranton, 1989; Cross, 1980; Rogers, 1989). Indeed, if a survey of literature on adult distance learners was done, a framework of these characteristics could easily be applied. A general belief about adult distance learners supported the idea that high motivation was a key to their success in anything from correspondence courses to Web-based videoconferencing. These distance learners were not the students who spent time on a typical college campus—not the typical students nursing would hope to attract to entry-level programs in 4-year colleges. Distance learners of this ilk seem to be those attracted to accelerated entry-level programs, in need of continuing education, or working professionals desiring advanced level education.

Convergence of Demographics, Motivation, and Barriers

Demographic Characteristics

A 1995 study by MacBrayne is applicable to one of the groups potentially attracted to nursing education. The demographic and motivational characteristics of 672 rural adult distance-education learners in an associate degree program were assessed by questionnaire. Of the 13 reasons listed for participating in distance education, course location and interest in the course content were cited by these learners as the most important. Other reasons in the top ten were the importance of the course for a future career and the desire to obtain a degree (MacBrayne, 1995). Applying the framework of characteristics of adult learners, there is a match between the framework and motivational qualities: degree seeking, information seeking, attaining goals, and enhancement of job ability (MacBrayne,

1995). As Knowles (1970) points out, these characteristics are also what make adults different from children when coming to an educational experience. These motivational qualities are not unique to the distance education venue; they can be seen in adult learners on campus.

Rossman (1993) indicates that students engaged in distance education are not typical of adolescents going to college on a residential campus. As more mature and self-disciplined students, distance learners already had some college experience and sought distance education courses either to accelerate or finish their undergraduate education (Rossman, 1993). A further characteristic noted by both Rossman and MacBrayne (1995) was that most of the participants were female. In Rossman's study, two thirds of the participants were female and cited unaffordable or inadequate childcare as reasons for participating in distance education.

Barriers

Barriers to typical educational activities are often the motivators for participating in distance education. Lack of time, cost, home responsibilities, job responsibilities, lack of self-confidence, and lack of interest often lead students to seek distance education activities (Cardenas, 2000; Hyatt, 1992; MacBrayne, 1995). Learners who perceive these barriers to their continued education often find that the control of time, place, and pace of education offered by distance education is extremely attractive (Wallace, 1996). Adults who claim they are too old to learn or who dislike the idea of group work in organized, on-campus classes are drawn to the independent and solitary nature of distance education opportunities. Those who lack confidence in their own abilities either to finish a course or keep up in the course are also drawn to this venue (Grace, 1994).

Although it is clear that there are demonstrated differences between distance learners and traditional students in their reasons for engagement, it is also clear that there are significant differences in their perceived barriers and motivators in distance education. Typical adolescents have no issues with being too old to learn. They may be too busy partying to learn, but rarely perceive themselves as incapable of learning. They also do not usually have barriers to learning such as childcare, job, and family issues. It would seem that their participation in distance education activities would be minimal. Yet, recent research shows that younger students are also taking advantage of distance education courses. These "second-generation" distance learners are also drawn to this venue. What is their motivation for taking advantage of distance education opportunities on a residential campus? What motivates them to start, continue, and complete those classes?

CURRENT DISTANCE EDUCATION STUDENTS: A SURPRISING FINDING

Study Background

Much research has been devoted to the highly motivated, mature student who participates in distance education activities. However, a study by Qureshi, Morton, and Antosz in 2002 demonstrated a surprising twist on the characteristics of distance learners. In survey research at a Canadian university, 120 distance learners and 120 on-campus students (the control group) were randomly selected to participate; 174 respondents (79 distance learners) answered a questionnaire designed to assess demographic characteristics, experience related to computer skills, motivation to enroll in distance or on-campus courses, and barriers to education (Qureshi et al., 2002). Four models corresponding to the framework seen in previous studies of the more mature learner were examined: a demographic model, an experiential model, a motivational model, and an inhibitory model (Qureshi et al., 2002). The experiential model that examined previous distance education and computer experience was not studied in previous research on distance education.

The Models

Demographic Model

Statistics in the demographic model demonstrated that distance learners were more likely to have children, have higher incomes, and be in a higher year of their undergraduate program. Based on previous studies of distance learners noted earlier, this was a consistent finding (MacBrayne, 1995; Wallace, 1996). The age of this group of students, both distance and on-campus, was younger than most previous studies of distance education: 42% of the students were ages 20 to 24, and 33.9% of the students were younger than 20. A shift in the demographics of current distance learners is distinct.

Inhibitory Model

Barriers to distance education were examined in the inhibitory model. Findings were consistent with previous educational studies (Cardenas, 2000; Hyatt, 1992; MacBrayne, 1995) and demonstrated that individual life situations, the dispositions of the learner, and institutional barriers such as location of the campus were of more concern to distance students than to on-campus students. Learning styles of the students within the two groups was not significant.

Motivational Model

It was in the motivational model that disparate statistics were found. Variables within this model included acquire knowledge, personal gain, meet community goals, social reasons, escape a situation, fulfill obligations, personal fulfillment, and gain cultural knowledge (Qureshi et al., 2001). A majority of the variables clearly supported differences between the distance and on-campus groups, supporting the idea that motivation is also different between the groups. Although that finding is not questionable, what is surprisingly questionable is that the on-campus group appeared more highly motivated than the distance education group. This finding is in direct opposition to notions from previous studies (Parrott, 1995; Willis, 2002) and andragogical theory (Knowles, 1978) that distance learners were more motivated.

Implications of the Study

Although the barriers and demographics of this current group were similar when compared to the existing framework of characteristics of distance learners, current distance education students were shown to be less motivated than their counterparts in previous studies and less motivated than their counterparts on campus. Several explanations for this surprising finding were put forth by the authors. The proliferation of high technology within Web-based courses might make the courses appear easier and thus more appealing to less motivated learners (Qureshi et al., 2001). Learners with multiple conflicts between family, job, and education might choose the course that seems easier because achievement would be enhanced. Another explanation by the authors has to do with the value of peer-to-peer experience or the value of an audience for the on-campus learners. Perhaps this characteristic of the classroom experience appeals less to the distance learner, who is typically independent and solitary. Thus, the distance learner wants to complete the course work as quickly as possible, feeling that doing it themselves is better than doing it with a group. Whether this is indicative of low motivation or is simply an uncharted characteristic of newer distance learners is a subject for further research.

HOW TO MAKE IT MATTER

The varying studies about the differences in the demographics and motivation levels of distance education students perhaps pose more questions about motivation than they answer. A dichotomy appears to exist between distance learners of the past and current distance learners. Distance learners of the past were older and appeared to be more motivated than their counterparts on campus. Today's distance learners seem to be younger and less motivated than their counterparts on campus. What is clear from an examination of both groups of learners is their willingness to engage in the process of education if they perceive a payoff in some form or another. This extrinsic motivation that Zull (2002) discusses does indeed lead to some of these learners becoming intrinsically motivated. What remains unclear from an examination of these groups of learners is exactly what motivates them to continue the educational endeavor once they have started. Once you engage them, how do you keep them? But—and this is the larger question—how do we accomplish that? Recent studies of varying types of distance learners provide some guidance.

Interaction and the Efficacy of Distance Education

Holmberg (1983) and Moore (1989) postulated that interactions between learners and their peers and learners and their instructors could be possible predictors for motivation in distance learning. Holmberg's contention that students learn by engaging in guided didactic conversations with faculty members applied primarily to formal classroom instruction. These conversations assisted in the development of a personal relationship between student and instructor that in turn created increased motivation in the students and enhanced learning outcomes (Holmberg, 1983). In 1995, Holmberg presented a theory of distance education that was based on his 1983 work on didactic conversations. Seven postulates were delineated:

> 1) feelings of personal relations between the instructor and student to promote study pleasure and motivation; 2) that such feelings would be supported by well-developed instructional materials and two-way communications; 3) that study motivation was important for the attainment of study goals; 4) that the atmosphere of friendly conversation favors feelings of personal relation according to postulate 1; 5) that communications within natural conversation are easily understood and remembered; 6) that the conversation concept can be successfully translated for use by the media available to distance students; and that 7) planning and guiding the curriculum were necessary for organized study at a distance. (Holmberg, 1995, p. 47)

Moore included interactions with multiple entities within the learning community in the distance education endeavor. Interactions certainly were between student and instructor, but also between students and other students and between students and the course content. Interactions within this model are multidirectional and built on reciprocity among all participants and the course content (Moore, 1989). This latter interaction between course content and learner includes two subcategories: interaction between the learner and inanimate learning resources such as books, tapes, and articles; and interaction between the learner and the interface to the technology used to deliver the instruction (Hillman, Willis, & Gunawardena, 1994). Learner-learner interactions are the traditional small-group discussions, group projects, and group presentations. As in previous distance education studies, some students found this learner-learner interaction crucial to their success, while others did not (Biner, Welsh, Barone, Summers, & Dean, 1997).

Kelsey and D'souza (2004) conducted a study looking at the interactions in these three areas vital to distance education. Their findings may guide us in keeping students motivated once they make the commitment to take a distance education course.

Student-Instructor Interactions

Within the context of the student-instructor interactions, Kelsey and D'souza found that students were satisfied as long as they had telephone, e-mail, or face-to-face meetings with the instructor (2004). Online office hours and online synchronous discussions between faculty and student would fall into this same context. The key to continued motivation and success is frequent communication, the didactic conversation.

Student-Interface Interactions

The interaction of the students with course content is naturally dependent upon the technology used to deliver the content. The lower-level technologies of e-mail, Web sites, CD-ROMs, and videotapes consistently provided motivation for the students to engage in the material. Likewise, technologies such as Blackboard and WebCt, when fully functioning on a high-speed Internet connection, provided satisfaction and motivated the students to continue. Streaming video technologies and interactive videoconferencing fared less well due to their sophistication and problems with anything less than cable or DSL access to the Internet (Kelsey & D'souza, 2004).

Student-Student Interactions

Perhaps the most significant of the findings deals with the lack of importance of student-student interactions. Contrary to Moore's theory (1989), the majority of the students in the study did not demand this type of interaction, and many of the faculty members did not encourage it (Kelsey & D'souza, 2004). If this type of interaction were encouraged and as available as chat rooms, real-time discussions, and even face-to-face meetings, would the level of interest and motivation of the students' increase? Again, a question for future research.

CONCLUSION

In looking at the many facets of student motivation for distance learning, it is obvious that there is no one method for each type of student. Although the extrinsic motivation of many students is their first foray into distance education, subsequent journeys must be intrinsically motivated. What causes those students to become intrinsically motivated seems to be dependent on their demographics, their perceived barriers, their previous experience with distance education, and the importance of interactions among students, instructors, and the technology used to deliver the content.

Indeed, if nursing education sees distance education as a method to relieve the nursing shortage, increase the number of faculty, and plug the brain drain (AACN, 2000), then it must look at each group of learners on an individual basis and pay attention to the demographics, barriers, and interactions.

The high cost of developing and implementing a distance education program will be lost if students are not motivated to continue after a first course. Poor experiences with an initial venture into distance education can color the student's perspective of other distance courses as well as the educational endeavor as a whole.

It behooves us as educators to evaluate systematically the student group, the course offerings, and the interactive abilities of the faculty and students if we are to motivate our entry level, advanced level, and continuing-education–seeking nurses to continue using this mode of education.

REFERENCES

American Association of Colleges of Nursing. (2000a). *Distance learning is changing and challenging nursing education* [AACN issue bulletin]. Retrieved October 13, 2004, from www.aacn.nche.edu/Publications/issues/jan2000.htm

American Association of Colleges of Nursing. (2000b). *AACN white paper: Distance technology in nursing education.* Retrieved October 13, 2004, from www.aacn.nche.edu/Publications/positions/whitepaper.htm

Benshoff, J., & Lewis, H. (1992). *Nontraditional college students*. ERIC Clearing-house on Counseling and Personnel Services. Ann Arbor, MI: (ERIC Document Reproduction Service No. ED 347483). Retrieved September 29, 2004, from http://www.ed.gov/databases/ERIC_Digests/ed347483

Biner, P. M., Welsh, K. D., Barone, N. M., Summers, M., & Dean, R. S. (1997). The impact of remote-site group size on student satisfaction and relative performance in interactive telecourses. *American Journal of Distance Education, 11*(1), 22–33.

Cardenas, C. (2000, October). *Motivations for and barriers against participation in adult education. Leonardo project MOBA*. Paper presented at the Adult Education and the Labor Market VI Conference, Seville, Spain. Retrieved September 29, 2004, from www.evu.ruc.dk/eng/events/seville/moba.html

Chen, H. (1998). *Interaction in distance education*. Retrieved September 9, 2004, from http://seamonkey.ed.asu.edu/mcisaac/disted/week2

Cranton, P. (1989). *Planning instruction for adult learners*. Toronto, Canada: Wall and Emerson.

Cross, K. (1980). Our changing students and their impact on colleges: Prospects for a true learning society. *Phi Delta Kappan, 61*, 630–632.

Fraser, J., & Haughey, M. (1999). Administering student-related concerns in nursing distance education programs. *Journal of Distance Education, 14*(1). Retrieved October 13, 2004, from http://cade.athabascau.ca/vol14.1/fraser _et_al.html

Garland, M. R. (1994). The adult need for "personal control" provides a cogent guiding concept for distance education. *Journal of Distance Education, 19*(1). Retrieved October 13, 2004, from http://cade.athabascau.ca/vol19.1/garland. html

Grace, M. (1994). Meanings and motivations: Women's experiences of studying at a distance. *Open Education, 9*(1), 13–21.

Hillman, D. C. A., Willis, D. J., & Gunawardena, C. N. (1994). Learner-interface interaction in distance education: An extension of contemporary models and strategies for practitioners. *American Journal of Distance Education, 8*(2), 30–41.

Holmberg, B. (1983). Guided didactic conversation in distance education. In D. Sewart, D. Keegan, & B. Holmberg (Eds.), *Distance education: International perspectives* (pp. 114–122). New York: St. Martin's Press.

Holmberg, B. (1995). The evolution of the character and practice of distance education. *Open Learning, 10*(2), 47–53.

Howell, S. L., Williams, P. B., & Lindsay, N. K. (2003). Thirty-two trends affecting distance education: An informed foundation for strategic planning. *Online Journal of Distance Education Administration, 6*(3). Retrieved September 29, 2004, from www.westga.edu/~distance/ojdla/fall 63/howell63.html

Hyatt, S. (1992, May). *Developing and managing a multi-modal distance learning program in the two-year college*. Paper presented at the Annual International Conference of the National Institute for Staff and Organizational Development on Teaching Excellence and Conference of Administrators, Austin, TX (ED 349 068).

Kelsey, K. D., & D'souza, A. (2004). Student motivation for learning at a distance: Does interaction matter? *Online Journal of Distance Education Administration, 7*(2). Retrieved September 29, 2004, from www.westga.edu/%7Edistance/ojdla/summer72/kelsey.html

Knowles, M. S. (1970). *The modern practice of adult education: Andragogy versus pedagogy.* Chicago: Association Press/Follett.

Kohn, A. (1993). *Punished by rewards: The trouble with gold stars, incentive plans, A's, praise, and other bribes.* New York: Houghton Mifflin.

MacBrayne, P. (1995). Rural adults in community college distance education: What motivates them to enroll? In *New directions for community colleges* (pp. 85–93). San Francisco: Jossey-Bass.

Miller, M. D., Rainer, R. K., & Corley, J. K. (2003). Predictors of engagement and participation in an on-line course. *Online Journal of Distance Education Administration, 6*(3). Retrieved September 29, 2004, from www.westga.edu/%7Edistance/ojdla/spring61/miller61.html

Moore, M. G. (1989). Three types of interaction. *American Journal of Distance Education, 3*(2), 1–6.

Nichols, M. (2003). A theory for elearning. *Educational Technology and Society, 6*(2), 1–10.

Parrott, S. (1995). Future learning: Distance education in community colleges. ERIC Digest (ED385311). Available http://www.ed.gov/databases/ERIC_Digests/ed38511.html

Pintrich, P. R. (2003). A motivational science perspective on the role of student motivation in learning and teaching contexts. *Journal of Educational Psychology, 95,* 667–686.

Qureshi, E., Morton, L. L., & Antosz, E. (2002). An interesting profile–university students who take distance education courses show weaker motivation than on-campus students. *Online Journal of Distance Education Administration, 5*(4). Retrieved September 29, 2004, from www.westga.edu/~distance/ojdla/winter54/qureshi.html

Roberts, T. G., Irani, T., Lundy, L. K., & Telg, R. (2003, February). Institutional practices in evaluating distance education among agricultural institutions of higher learning. *Proceedings of the Southern Agricultural Education Research Conference,* Mobile, AL.

Rogers, A. (1989). *Teaching adults.* Philadelphia: Open University Press.

Rossman, P. (1993). *The emerging worldwide electronic university: Information age global higher education.* Westport, CT: Praeger.

Rovai, A. P., & Barnum, K. T. (2003). On-line course effectiveness: An analysis of student interactions and perceptions of learning. *Journal of Distance Education, 18*(1), 57–73.

Wallace, L. (1996). Changes in the demographics and motivations of distance education students. *Journal of Distance Education, 11*(1), 1–31.

Williams, P. E., & Hellman, C. M. (2004). Differences in self-regulation for online learning between first- and second-generation college students. *Research in Higher Education, 45*(1), 71–82.

Willis, B. (2002). Distance education at a glance: Guide #9. Retrieved September 29, 2004, from http://www.uidaho.edu/evo/dist9.html

Wolff, L. (2003). *Brain research, education, and technology.* Retrieved September 29, 2004, from www.TechKnowLogia.org

Zull, J. E. (2002). *The art of changing the brain: Enriching the practice of teaching by experiencing the biology of education.* Sterling, VA: Stylus.

CHAPTER 8

Online Learning as a Tool for Professional Development

Suzanne Hetzel Campbell

The American Nurses' Association (ANA) defines nurse professional development as "the lifelong process of active participation in learning activities to enhance professional practice" (Jackson, 2004). Nurses are challenged to maintain current knowledge on evidence-based professional practice and rapidly changing professional, ethical, and legal issues. Online education provides a means to enhance nursing professionals' clinical knowledge and skills, including technological, clinical decision making, leadership, management, even pharmaceutical advances and updates. This chapter will examine the use of online education as a viable tool for a variety of activities leading toward a nurse's professional development.

HEALTH PROFESSIONAL NEED
FOR CONTINUING EDUCATION

Nurses recognize the need for lifelong learning, and management acknowledges that environments rich in continuing education tend to advance staff development, increase morale, and promote retention (Postler-Slattery & Foley, 2003). In view of the present nursing shortage in all areas, as well as the constantly shifting health care setting, new illnesses, and changing patient responses to drugs, infections, and the environment, the challenge is to provide continuing education to all nurses. This education must take into consideration the complexity of the staff's varying backgrounds, certification, and interest, as well as the limited resources provided for professional development.

Access to and use of online continuing education by physicians and nurses have been studied (Casebeer, Bennett, Kristofeo, Carillo, & Centor, 2002; Cobb, 2003; Cobb & Baird, 1999). Findings indicate that the use of the Internet for professional development among physicians and nurses is growing, especially in relationship to continuing education. However, easy access to relevant and credible information that is quickly available, easy to use, and relatively low cost were priorities identified by health professionals (Cobb, 2003). In addition, indexing the clinically focused health information online is challenging but important to enhance its usefulness to nurses and other health care providers (Casebeer et al., 2002).

Research on Health Professionals' Use of the Internet for Health Information

Several studies have been done examining health professionals' use of the Internet for health information and continuing education. Overall, the studies' results provide limited generalizable information because they are geographically limited and have low response rates. They report conflicting findings and emphasize the need for further research.

One of the more thorough and informative studies, a randomized market survey of 800 occupational health and safety professionals in an eight-state Midwest region of the United States, found that 87.4% reported a high likeliness to participate in continuing education (CE) or advanced degrees via the Internet; 79% did not feel being on campus was important; and 68% were reimbursed for continuing education costs (Carlson & Olson, 2001). However, this study failed to focus on nursing professionals while Lathey and Hodge (2001) surveyed 600 occupational health nurses in New York State and obtained a 28% response rate ($N = 165$), finding that 38% used the Internet to gather health information and 65% were interested in continuing education via the Internet.

In contrast, Hegge, Powers, Hendrick, and Vinson (2002) found that less than 50% of registered nurses surveyed in South Dakota felt their continuing education needs were met by the Internet. Although 75% had computers at home and 76% had computers at work, less than 20% of registered nurses used the computer for continuing education (Hegge et al., 2002). Finally, a survey of Nevada Advanced Practice Nurses (APNs), found the most frequently used form of continuing education was in-person conferences and the least preferred form was live-satellite conferences. Their top three preferences for continuing education were (a) in-person conference, (b) print-based self-study, and (c) interactive video conference. In conclusion, this study found that the computer-based modes for continuing education including the Internet and CD-ROMs, were among the least used by Nevada APNs (Charles & Mamary, 2002).

Despite the results of these studies, little data exist related to computer use by nurses for obtaining professional development and accessing continuing education opportunities. The variety of programs available suggests this form of continuing education is more widely used than demonstrated by the above surveys, especially recently.

Present Examples of Professional Development through Web-Based Education in Nursing

The Internet has made Web-based education feasible for those involved in a variety of professions. In nursing, refresher courses have been designed via the Internet to address the nursing shortage and get nurses to return to the workforce (White, Roberts, & Brannan, 2003). The authors describe how collaborative distance education using a Web-based instructional design answers some of the problems of cost, effectiveness, and access for nursing refresher courses (White et al., 2003).

Career mobility is another educational issue that is sparking interest in online education. RN to BSN programs have begun migrating to the Web, offering the advantages of interactive opportunities, resources on the Internet, and flexible, cost-effective, and easily accessible alternatives to traditional education. For nurses juggling work, family responsibilities, care of aging parents, and other life stressors, this is a feasible option for professional development (O'Brien & Renner, 2000; Zucker & Asselin, 2003).

Another use of Web-based education is for professional development toward an advanced degree, such as a nurse practitioner degree. Graduate classes are offered online and include core courses like pharmacology (Bata-Jones & Avery, 2004) and pathophysiology (Yucha & Princen, 2000), as well as modules specific to cultural assessment (Clark & Thornam, 2002) and pediatric health assessment (Kieckhefer, Stevens, & Frkonja, 2002). Three modules were created for a nurse practitioner program and they utilized an interactive framework that used Web links and realistic self-studies resembling clinical practice. Registration was accomplished online and pre- and posttesting allowed evaluation of learning (Hayes, Huckstadt, & Gibson, 2000).

Finally, Web-based continuing education has been used to offer specialty-specific information in the form of summer- and semester-long institutes, like the Web-based Genetics Institute for a Nursing Audience (Prows, Hetteberg, Hopkin, Latta, & Powers, 2004).

RN Needs for Online Education

A study using focus groups of RNs at a military hospital identified five themes related to the need for professional development. The thematic groupings included (1) specific development needs for leadership, clinical/specialty practice, competence development, and maintenance, (2) methods to provide continuing education, (3) methods to evaluate the effectiveness and efficiency of continuing education, (4) barriers to development, and (5) professional development issues impacting retention specific to military nurses (Bibb et al., 2003).

The themes described in the Bibb et al. (2003) study focus on professional development and continuing education. Specific needs for new clinical skills and current evidence-based practice information exist in all specialty areas of nursing. Pharmaceutical updates can be provided via the Internet in online continuing-education self-study modules. Unique case studies allow opportunities for collaboration and professional development. So with the increasing needs for continuing education, why is obtaining it such a challenge for RNs?

ADVANTAGES OF ONLINE EDUCATION

For RNs, shift work, high patient acuity, and unpredictable patient flow all create barriers to attending continuing education programs (Curran-Smith & Best, 2004). Benefits of online education include its accessibility and flexibility. The opportunities for professional development include career advancement such as course work toward certification or to prepare for certification exams; contact hours for participation; or as a means for career advancement (RN to BSN–clinical ladders). Web-based education can help RNs maintain evidence-based practice knowledge and skills. In addition, overburdened practitioners can more realistically spare time for a 30-minute online course versus a full day or weekend conference.

Another barrier of traditional continuing education involves the cost that can include travel, lodging, food, and registration. Costs should be lower for a Web-based program, depending on who is offering the program. Web-based instruction developed by pharmaceutical companies or as the result of a federal or private grant may be free to participants.

Nursing managers also have difficulty accessing continuing education. The development of educational resources and support for leadership and management is viable via online methods. Providing interactive workshops presenting information focused on enhancing knowledge and skills is feasible. Finally, creating an arena for discussion and support for practitioners via Web-based education can lead to interdisciplinary collaboration and knowledge development.

Finally, for some areas, continuing education is geographically inaccessible. Online education can reach rural areas that may lack resources and access to current continuing education. Clinics caring for underserved populations may be more easily reached via the Internet, as long as they have Internet and computer resources.

POTENTIAL BARRIERS OF ONLINE CONTINUING EDUCATION

Barriers unique to the Web-based education programs include access to computers and the Internet, especially in developing countries, and attitudes toward learning via the World Wide Web (Cragg, Edwards, Yue, Xin, & Hui, 2003; Curran-Smith & Best, 2004). Another potential barrier is the need for new skill sets for online learning technologies for both learners and educators. Computer literacy among faculty and staff is an important consideration when developing and implementing online education. Faculty must learn to present the content, assist students in applying the knowledge, establish a shared understanding, and identify opportunities for improved communication (Curran-Smith & Best, 2004).

For continuing education, the administrative logistics are substantial, and online education is not an exception. Finding staff time to complete the programs or attend the live satellite teleconferencing programs is a management issue. How is time and money budgeted for staff to attend continuing education? Who is encouraged to participate in professional development programs and how frequently? Are staffs rewarded for attending continuing education? Hospitals have initiated programs to provide staff incentive, such as "accruing" points by taking advantage of self-directed learning opportunities, which will lead to off-site educational programs (Reed, 1999). Others have mandated continuing education by including it in job descriptions and performance appraisals (Postler-Slattery & Foley, 2003). Similar techniques may be used to encourage online courses for staff development.

With the busy lifestyles of nursing professionals, allocating a set day, time, and appropriate environment is important in keeping to the commitment for professional development. Utilizing the Internet in a library, private office, or meeting room would be more successful than using a computer in the midst of a busy workstation where phone, patient, and staff interruptions are likely. Having technology available is necessary, as well as less technically dependent back-up methods for periodic system glitches or crashes. This includes technological support for those participating in the program.

As with any continuing education program, verifying the following is important: that the continuing education provider is accredited with a good reputation, the content describes expected outcomes and logical and attainable objectives are outlined, and the program fits RNs' needs (Jackson, 2004). In the case of those supported by pharmaceutical or market-based companies, one should also evaluate the program for bias and examine the faculty disclosure statements.

It is suggested that the workload, attrition and failure rates for online courses are greater (Sapp & Simon, in press), but no one has examined continuing education programs in these areas. With proper computer skills, commitment of individual time, and evaluation of the online program, the learning environment can be as successful as any other.

METHODOLOGIES FOR ONLINE LEARNING

The variety of settings and practice specialties in nursing creates a need for culturally appropriate, setting- and specialty-focused information. Areas of concentration may include, but are not limited to, technology, clinical skills, and interventions for client symptom and disease management, as well as issues related to administrative and leadership responsibilities. Web-based education and online learning opportunities have the potential to meet this need.

An array of methods to provide this education exists, including varied materials, teaching formats, and techniques of presentation. Materials can be text based, in the form of PowerPoint slides or lecture dialogue. Pre- and posttests can be used for the provision of continuing education units or contact hours and to evaluate participant learning. Video clips can provide demonstration of specific assessments or skills and allow for vicarious experiences and participant learning through role modeling.

Interactive exercises such as matching, short answer, or crossword puzzles can enhance learning by providing immediate feedback. Web-based education can utilize simulations and progressive problem solving to improve critical thinking skills.

In addition to a variety of materials, teaching formats can vary as well. Teaching formats include a single presenter to an audience that may or may not be able to interact, the use of case studies to provide real-life scenarios for learning, or discussion threads that are recorded over time and used for learning. Case studies can be presented to provide clinically focused content; Internet resources of Web links can provide important information for future reference and use.

Presentation of information for professional development may be via teleconferencing in a myriad of formats. The teleconference may be live and displayed to a live audience; it may be presented in video or audio format, or both. In addition, the teleconference may be archived and available to participants in video and audio format with other presentation materials, for example, handouts, PowerPoint slides, and CD-ROMs. Depending on the style of presentation, interaction may be live, such as a videoconference where the presenter can see participants via cameras and answer questions while presenting. By contrast, in an audio format, where participants are also linked via the Internet in a meeting session, individuals are able to ask questions by typing or calling them into the live session.

Location of the attendees is determined by participant needs and technological availability. When participants attend at the actual time the presentation is given, they can be gathered in a large auditorium, observing and participating in the presentation as a group. In contrast, a smaller group of attendees at a local clinic or physician's office can attend the live teleconference. Finally, individuals may attend from the comfort of their own offices or homes, in live time or as part of the archived recording of the teleconference. Self-study text-based, case-study–based, or individual learning modules are usually done at the participant's convenience. However, reimbursement for time spent on continuing education remains an unresolved issue.

Web-based education has the potential to provide a variety of materials, teaching formats, and methods of presentation. It can consider the values and beliefs of diverse underserved populations cared for by local community and hospital health centers, federal and state health programs, and physician offices. Programs may serve practitioners as well as students, academics, researchers, and administrators. The opportunities for professional development and career advancement using online education are limitless.

CONCLUSIONS

There are definitely challenges to be overcome in relation to online education. Increased demand from the new generation of health care professionals will necessitate more options and increased availability of Web-based continued education programs. Federal support is in place for the development of programs for distance education for many health professionals. Issues of computer literacy and availability, technological support and consistency, and learner/educator attitude toward online educational methodology will determine the success and participant satisfaction with this form of continuing education.

REFERENCES

Bata-Jones, B., & Avery, M. D. (2004). Teaching pharmacology to graduate nursing students: Evaluation and comparison of Web-based and face-to-face methods. *Journal of Nursing Education, 43,* 185–189.

Bibb, S., Malebranche, M., Crowell, D., Altman, C., Lyon, S., Carlson, A., et al. (2003). Professional development needs of registered nurses practicing at a military community hospital. *Journal of Continuing Education in Nursing, 34*(1), 39–45.

Carlson, V., & Olson, D. (2001). Technology-enhanced learning/distance education: Market survey of occupational health and safety professionals. *American Industrial Hygiene Association Journal, 62,* 349–355.

Casebeer, L., Bennett, N., Kristofeo, R., Carillo, A., & Centor, R. (2002). Physician Internet medical information seeking and online continuing education use patterns. *Journal of Continuing Education in the Health Professions, 22*(1), 33–42.

Charles, P., & Mamary, E. (2002). New choices for continuing education: A statewide survey of the practices and preferences of nurse practitioners. *Journal of Continuing Education in Nursing, 33*(2), 88–91.

Clark, L., & Thornam, C. (2002). Using educational technology to teach cultural assessment. *Journal of Nursing Education, 41,* 117–120.

Cobb, S. (2003). Comparison of oncology nurse and physician use of the Internet for continuing education. *Journal of Continuing Education in Nursing, 34,* 184–188.

Cobb, S., & Baird, S. (1999). Oncology nurses' use of the Internet for continuing education: A survey of Oncology Nursing Society Congress attendees. *Journal of Continuing Education in Nursing, 30,* 199–202.

Cragg, C., Edwards, N., Yue, Z., Xin, S., & Hui, Z. (2003). Integrating Web-based technology into distance education for nurses in China: Computer and Internet access and attitudes. *CIN: Computers, Informatics, Nursing, 21,* 265–274.

Curran-Smith, J., & Best, S. (2004). An experience with an online learning environment to support a change in practice in an emergency department. *CIN: Computers, Informatics, Nursing, 22,* 107–110.

Hayes, K., Huckstadt, A., & Gibson, R. (2000). Developing interactive continuing education on the Web. *Journal of Continuing Education in Nursing, 31,* 199–203.

Hegge, M., Powers, P., Hendrick, L., & Vinson, J. (2002). Competence, continuing education, and computers. *Journal of Continuing Education in Nursing, 33*(1), 24.

Jackson, R. (2004). In hot pursuit of higher learning. *Nursing Management, 35,* 13.

Kieckhefer, G., Stevens, A., & Frkonja, J. (2002). Teaching pediatric health assessment: using Internet capabilities. *Journal of Pediatric Health Care, 16,* 180–186.

Lathey, J., & Hodge, B. (2001). Information seeking behavior of occupational health nurses: How nurses keep current with health information. *American Association of Occupational Health Nurses Journal, 49*(2), 87–95.

O'Brien, B., & Renner, A. (2000). Nurses online: Career mobility for registered nurses. *Journal of Professional Nursing, 16*(1), 13–20.

Postler-Slattery, D., & Foley, K. (2003). The fruits of lifelong learning. *Nursing Management, 34*(2 pt. 1), 34–37.

Prows, C. A., Hetteberg, C., Hopkin, R. J., Latta, K. K., & Powers, S. M. (2004). Development of a Web-based genetics institute for a nursing audience. *Journal of Continuing Education in Nursing, 35,* 223–231.

Reed, M. K. (1999). Empowering lifelong learners. *Nursing Management, 30*(4), 48.

Sapp, D. A., & Simon, J. (in press). Comparing grades in online and face-to-face writing courses: Interpersonal accountability and institutional commitment. *Computers and Composition.*

White, A., Roberts, V., & Brannan, J. (2003). Returning nurses to the workforce: Developing an online refresher course. *Journal of Continuing Education in Nursing, 34*(2), 59–63.

Yucha, C., & Princen, T. (2000). Insights learned from teaching pathophysiology on the World Wide Web. *Journal of Nursing Education, 39*(2), 68–72.

Zucker, D. M., & Asselin, M. (2003). Migrating to the Web: The transformation of a traditional RN to BS program. *Journal of Continuing Education in Nursing, 24*(2), 86–89.

PART 2

Experiences of Specific Programs

Teaching Online Pathophysiology: The University of Colorado Health Science Center School of Nursing

Haeok Lee, Nancy Holloway, and Leeann Field

This course is designed for nurses who are experienced in the management of pathophysiologic disorders. It includes advanced concepts in pathophysiologic principles, using a systems approach to provide understanding of the dynamic aspects of disease and disease processes, and foundation for assessment and management of the acutely or chronically ill client. Epidemiology, etiology, life span, cultural concepts, diagnostic reasoning, and current research findings are integrated into select content areas.

INSTITUTIONAL INFRASTRUCTURE AND SUPPORT

The teaching and learning process of an online pathophysiology course begins by looking first at the infrastructure and support for online education at the institutional level.

What equipment is necessary for faculty and students?

What is the plan for upgrades (hardware and software)?

What levels and types of technical support, education, and training are in place for faculty and students?

What other basic support systems (e.g., online registration, access to grades online, or access to library journal articles) need to be in place for online learners, learners who may never set foot on campus?

Who develops and supports these systems and how do they integrate with the online learning environment?

What basic computer skills and knowledge do students and faculty need in order to be successful learners and teachers in an online course?

What additional special skills do they need to know and practice in order to continue successfully within your institution?

With regard to these skills, if student or faculty skills are below the basic levels needed, or if they do not possess the special skills, what responsibility does your institution want to take in order to bring them up to speed in acceptable skill and knowledge levels?

Will you serve the entire student population with the support structures, convenient features, and useful tools that are in place for online students?

How do online courses interface with your institution's information systems (IS), registration, and so forth?

How will the faculty and students come to know the answers to all these questions?

Much more is involved than just deciding to teach a basic science course online. The development of the course alone is one giant hurdle in itself, but so many other issues and answers need to be defined and examined before the course development even begins. The answers to the above questions have a significant impact on how and what you do when developing your course. A brief examination of what the School of Nursing (SON) at University of Colorado Health Sciences Center (UCHSC) did regarding these questions will give you some insight into how these efforts helped lay the foundation for creating and teaching an online pathophysiology course.

Generally, all the faculty at the SON are provided with an office, a computer, additional computer storage space on a network drive that is backed up daily, an e-mail account, and an Internet connection that is accessible to the entire campus as well as remotely from home computers. Computers run on a Windows-based operating system and the Microsoft Office Suite software products installed on every computer. Many of these decisions were already determined for the school at a campus level through the IS department. The budget, software licensing agreements, and plans for continual upgrades of technology are directed from the main IS office, and implementation efforts are carried out on an individual school level by the school's IS personnel, who work as liaisons with the campus's central IS department.

Students who contemplate applying to the university are made aware via marketing and application materials that they need to own, acquire, or have access to their own personal computer (PC), desktop or laptop, upon attending this institution. Materials available indicate minimum hardware and software requirements for their PCs. Students are responsible for complying with these minimum specifications and carry the burden of this expense. Students who are accepted and register for courses receive a student e-mail account and have Internet access through a local dial-up phone number. Those students who are not local to the school are encouraged to secure another Internet service provider (ISP), to avoid incurring long-distance telephone charges. Training for using e-mail, the Internet, search engines, and databases is provided on a campus level to all students through the campus library, but mostly through online self-paced tutorials. However, some face-to-face (F2F) classes are offered. Students also have access to free virus protection software for their PCs and regular upgrades to the software as long as they are students.

UCHSC SON has established infrastructure, the Office of Online Education Services (OOES). This office is staffed with an instructional designer, a Web administrator, a programmer, and an administrative assistant. The personnel in this office developed *Online Central!*, a Web page built into the SON Web site (see side note). This central resource page supports online learning throughout the SON.

First-time online students at the SON are directed to click the Getting Started Checklist. This list takes students through a series of 12 items to see if they are ready to begin their online education at UCHSC SON. Clicking yes to an item in the checklist indicates that students know the information and should proceed to the next item on the list. Clicking no to an item on the list launches students into a new Web window that provides information to aid them in their knowledge deficit.

First-time faculty who are teaching or developing online courses are directed to click the Faculty Resources link. This link gives access to a number of resources to aid faculty in developing and teaching endeavors. In particular, they have access to the *Faculty Handbook for Building*

Online Central!

Getting Started Checklist

Access My Online Course

FAQs

Course Schedules

Student Technology

Hardware & Software Requirements for Online Students

Course and Instructor Evaluations

Technical Support

Denison Library

UCHSC Book Store

Faculty Resources

Suggestion Box

Online Courses, with updates on OOES process and procedures, instructional design strategies, best practices for teaching, and tips for writing in an online environment.

Faculty and students are also required to complete a prerequisite course called Online Course Skills before teaching or registering for an online course. The design of this course gives students and faculty their first insight into the look and feel of an SON online course. Passing this course provides foundational knowledge and skills to enable them to be successful in their online courses at the SON.

THEORETICAL BACKGROUND

Human-technology interaction (HTI) comprised of this online pathophysiology course is designed and based on the construct of social presence, which directly affect the user-technology relationship. A successful interactive online pathophysiology, based on educative HTI, supports and encourages the social aspects of learning. This section will discuss social presence and its role in learning.

Short, Williams, and Christie (1976) stated that all situations involve communication, and each situation places unique controls on how written, verbal, and nonverbal cues are utilized: computer-mediated communication (CMC) is no different. Scholars in psychology and CMC refer to the *quality* of the medium of communication and the *quality* of the relationship as "social presence" (Gunawardena, 1995; Gunawardena & Zittle, 1997; Short et al., 1976). Any medium of communication that is gauged as "being warm, personal, sensitive and sociable" has the highest degree of social presence (Short et al., 1976, p. 66). In addition, Short et al. hypothesized that verbal and nonverbal cues are such vital components to establishing intimacy and immediacy in communication that people will find a way to express them regardless of the type of medium utilized. Therefore, social presence in a CMC environment for this online pathophysiology course is created by operationalizing intimacy and immediacy into the course design.

Intimacy is the perception of physical closeness or familiarization among the participants in a communication presence. The factors of intimacy in face-to-face communication are physical distance, eye contact, smiling, and personal topics of conversation (Short et al., 1976, p. 72); however, for this online course, we developed several strategies to create and foster the perception of intimacy and immediacy for both the learner and educator. First, we pay attention in providing students with built-in time for socialization and create a safe place to discuss individual and group assignments. Second, we provide private and public forums where they can air their frustrations. Third, we provide certain behaviors such as role modeling, participating dialogue, and attention to netiquette to provide other group members with personal information of their choosing. Fourth, we emphasize the use of informal language in text, saving formal language for assignments. Immediacy is the perceived emotional and time distance between the instructor and the students. Written texture or visual cues were utilized to foster immediacy such as preprogrammed feedback design, allowing us to provide correct answers in real time at the submission of students' answers to the quizzes; a variety of asynchronous forums and synchronous chat rooms were included in the design to foster the perception of immediacy.

The lack of verbal and visual cues may not foster immediacy and intimacy, because users can gauge the authenticity of the other and the ensuing relationships without the challenge of stereotypical characteristics (Holloway, 2000; Tanis, 2003). Social presence is fostered and nurtured in computer-mediated online education, and is leading to the development of successful human-technology interaction in this online pathophysiology course.

COURSE DESIGN

The focus of this course is to educate students rather than to present information. The curriculum is competency-based, where prior learning is assessed and validated and the development of skills promotes each student's success. The role of the instructor is not just to provide information, but also to facilitate the self and group learning process, as well as to evaluate the learning experiences. The concepts of immediacy and intimacy were embedded in the pathophysiology course during the design phase, by utilizing standardized template texture modules as well as multiple images in the design phase, with close collaboration between the educator and online education design team.

Using a Standardized Template

Faculty is also required to use standard icons for all basic features offered in WebCT. For example, all courses use the same icon for the syllabus, modules, conference center (WebCT's bulletin board feature—asynchronous communication), student presentation area (a file-sharing area), chat (real time—synchronous communication), WebCT's Internal Course e-mail feature, calendar, assignment box, white board, quizzes/exams, and final course evaluations. We also use the same template to develop the syllabus for this online course. Though you may think that these types of standards stifle imagination and creativity for courses, students in particular find it very refreshing to go into every SON online course and immediately be familiar with the lay of the land for every course. Not having to navigate or learn a different look and feel based on the individual preferences of instructors proves to be a convenient, timesaving mechanism—in other terms, *immediacy* perception—in delivering our courses. Both students and faculty immediately know where and how to find the information and tools they need; they can hit the ground running, to coin an old phrase.

A typical course home page, Advanced Pathophysiology, for example, has a universal icon for the following:

- The syllabus (which contains the course description, course outcome competencies or objectives, information about the instructor and his or her contact information—e-mail, phone numbers, office hours, etc.—course text and/or readings, the schedule, evaluations and grading, and policies)

- Modules/Units

- Conference Center (a bulletin board designed to permit the asynchronous)

- Chat Room (for synchronous interaction, if desired)

- WebCT's e-mail

- Student Presentation Area

- Quizzes/Exam (not all courses have quizzes or exams)

- Online Grade Book

- Student Evaluation of the Course (visible and available to the students during the last week of the course)

Because icons are standard in all online courses and the use of these icons has already been introduced to students through the Online Course Skills, students quickly know exactly which icon to select based on their initial or current needs.

Using Texture for Modules (Units)

A total of 15 topic areas comprising a module (unit) are developed based on the required textbook. They include basic mechanism of disease, tumor/carcinogenesis, the immune response, and selected disorders of the following systems: cardiovascular, respiratory, hematologic, neuralgic, endocrine, urinary, digestive, musculoskeletal, and reproductive. The concepts of texture and social presence work in concert to enhance the course. Each module is summarized by combining the tone of casual conversation and technological language, which brings the learner closer to the information (intimacy) as opposed to formal (textbook) language, which distances students. The use of pronouns and contractions (immediacy) kept the language casual; it was important to keep informal language style consistent throughout the modules. The units are summarized in the tutorial by way of presentation style. Five to 10 quizzes made up of critical thinking questions are in the content of each unit (see more information under Competency Evaluation in this chapter).

Images

A Web site link is inside the content of each unit. The Web site used most often is http://www-medlib.med.utah.edu/WebPath/webpath.html# MENU, which was developed in 1994 by Dr. Edward Klatt of the Department of Pathology at the University of Utah. These materials are available through the Web site or by purchasing a CD individually or instructionally. Web sources include more than 1,900 images, including text, a tutorial, a laboratory exercise, and examination items for self-assessment that demonstrate broad and general microscopic pathologic findings associated with the 15 topic areas. Visual knowledge-based presentations are available for viewing the images of the pathophysiology concept to illustrate the basic mechanism of disease, which is described in the text. Each section consists of a series of images demonstrating microscopic pathologic findings, some diagrams, and a short description of each image.

ONLINE TEACHING-LEARNING PROCESS

This course uses collaborative technologies, including a course Web site, e-mail, communication, and Internet-based information to enhance learning, increase communication, and engage the geographically dispersed participant. The course Web site includes course information such as syllabus, schedule, and information about the instructor, student biosketches, e-mail, and phone numbers. A conference center was designed to permit the asynchronous student, or student and faculty with student interaction in a chat room for synchronous interaction (if desired), a student presentation area for student projects, and hyperlinks to the school library and the World Wide Web.

The purpose of the conference center is for central posting responses regarding each unit's assignments and for participant/instructor discussion and communication. Participants call each other by first name or by individually identified nicknames and make liberal use of emoticons and informal language in discussion areas, with formal language reserved for presentations and assignment completion. A variety of asynchronous forums and synchronous chat rooms contributed to intimacy and immediacy because synchronous chat allows for spontaneous conversation and asynchronous communication encourages reflective thought. Course and student e-mail systems and individual contact information contributed to the sense of intimacy among participants and fostered immediacy between students and course educators. Case studies directed the students to apply educative resources to their respective clinical interests and thus provided immediacy by decreasing the distance between theory and practice. The critical thinking questions and online exams promoted immediacy by providing instantaneous feedback to the students about their educative process and to the educators about the students' course status.

Typically, on the first day of the week the instructor posts introductory information on the week's topic and confirms all assignments, such as readings from the textbook, completing a case study, or preparing a paper on the topic identified in the course's module for that week. The instructor may also direct students to other helpful URLs, post an addendum or short lecture applicable to that week's module or readings, elaborate on any of the material, and provide any supplemental information related to the topic that requires more explanation. Throughout the week, the student reads and works on assignments, as in a traditional classroom setting. The student uses the bulletin board to participate in class discussion, ask questions, and receive feedback. When assignments are due, students submit them online in a number of ways, according to the instructor's preference. Options include uploading a file to the student presentation area, posting to an assigned topic, attaching a file to a post in a topic, sending a WebCT e-mail, or attaching a file to a WebCT e-mail using WebCT's assignment box. After the instructor grades or reviews the assignment, the feedback and grade are sent back to students (usually by WebCT e-mail). Grades can also be posted to the student using WebCT's online gradebook feature.

COMPETENCY EVALUATION

This course has four prescribed outcome competencies. Course contents are tailored based on outcomes and therefore student and instructor expectation and preparation for this course are clear. The course evaluation was developed based on these outcome competencies as well, which are as follows:

1. Integrate assessment data and laboratory/diagnostic data to determine diagnostic probabilities.
2. Identify specific pathophysiologic processes, clinical manifestations, and system interactions of selected disease processes and disease states.
3. Demonstrate synthesis of advanced physiologic and pathophysiologic principles to the advanced practice nurse's role in assessment, diagnosis, planning, prevention, and patient teaching in diverse populations.
4. Evaluate current research findings in pathophysiology for relevancy and impact on nursing practice, including genetic and immunologic advances.

Competency evaluations are in three parts: (a) class participation including student's completion of critical thinking questions; (b) multiple-choice exams, and (c) case studies. Through reviewing critical thinking questions, case studies, and midterm exams, the instructor evaluates each student's progress and competencies in learning outcomes. Based on review and evaluation of student's competency, encouragement and feedback will be provided. Moreover, supplemental information either to clarify certain pathologic concepts or to correct misunderstandings is added through postings in the main communication channel known as the main forum.

The Purpose and Nature of Evaluation

Participation in Course Activities

This includes evidence of substantial reading, participation in group discussions, and contributions to the course Web site's conference center, as well as completion of critical thinking questions. There are 5 to 10 critical thinking questions in each unit to encourage the student to think and put the content together in an organized fashion. When the student answers these questions, the student can choose to view the instructor's answers. The critical thinking questions promoted immediacy by providing instantaneous feedback to students about their educative process and to the educators about the students' course status. The instructor monitors the student's answers, and if answers are in error in an area of concern, the instructor will intervene by posting supplemental information or will correct the problems. The critical thinking questions are used for evaluation of class participation purposes. Students are expected to complete these questions based on the course progression, which is an average of one unit per week. Based on the course progression, the instructor can monitor a student's progress.

Case Studies

For each of the modules, there are one or two case studies posted in the conference center. The case studies are developed to provide diverse experiences including age, gender, ethnicity, as well as acculturation. In the case study, there are lab findings, clinical symptoms and signs, and current and past medical histories. Students are asked to address the information presented in the actual case studies by assessing data, including laboratory/diagnostic and clinical information to make the nursing diagnosis, and a treatment plan that is threaded directly into the case study. Students also are asked to substantiate their assessment and treatment plan with current research findings to justify their decision in the nursing practice setting. Through the extensive use of case studies, the online pathophysiology course provides a venue for incorporating multiple diversity factors into the clinical management of pathophysiologic disorders. Netiquette and minimal use of slang help to prevent miscommunication among course participants. Case studies direct the students to apply educative resources to their respective clinical interests, and thus provide immediacy by decreasing the distance between theory and practice.

Midterm Examinations

The midterm exam is not just for evaluative purposes, but to provide learning experiences. For 2 days, the students are allowed to find answers by reading textbooks, journals, notes, course units, or by performing Internet searches. The searches are important, because many students who take an Internet course, particularly a pathophysiology course, have expressed anxiety about their learning progress, with questions such as how much do I have to know? Am I on the right path? How do I compare with other students in my class and in other institutions? Actually, this is a chance for students to apply their basic scientific knowledge of pathophysiology in their advanced practice while they are taking the midterm exam. However, the midterm exam is multiple-choice, and the questions are long. One third of the questions are in a short, case scenario style, and the students are asked to select a correct diagnosis, clinical signs and symptoms, and correct treatments, among other things. The online exams promoted immediacy by providing an instantaneous grade, as well as providing timely feedback to students about their level of learning process and to educators about the students' course status.

REFERENCES

Gunawardena, C. N. (1995). Social presence theory and implications for interaction and collaborative learning in computer conferences. *International Journal of Educational Telecommunications, 1*(2/3), 147–166.

Gunawardena, C. N., & Zittle, F. J. (1997). Social presence as a predictor of satisfaction within a computer-mediated conferencing environment. *American Journal of Distance Education, 11*(3), 8–26.

Holloway, N. (2000). *Social presence and nursing presence: An illuminating combination.* Unpublished manuscript.

Klatt, E. C. (1994). *Internet pathology laboratory for medical education.* Retrieved October 22, 2004, from http://www-medlib.med.utah.edu/WebPath/webpath.

Short, J., Williams, E., & Christie, B. (1976). *The social psychology of telecommunications*. London: Wiley.

Tanis, M. (2003). *Cues to identity in CMC. The impact on person perception and subsequent interaction outcomes*. (Master's thesis, University of Amsterdam). Enschede, Amsterdam: Print Partners Ipskamp.

CHAPTER 10

A Distance Learning Master's Degree Program for Nurse-Midwives and Nurse Practitioners: Frontier School of Midwifery and Family Nursing

Susan Stone

The purpose of this chapter is to provide an update on the progress of the development of an innovative distance-education program for nurse-midwives and nurse practitioners at the Frontier School of Midwifery and Family Nursing. The establishment, early development, and operation of the Community-Based Nurse-midwifery Education Program (CNEP) were described in an earlier edition of this book (Stone, Ernst, & Shaffer, 2000).

BACKGROUND

The Frontier School of Midwifery and Family Nursing (FSMFN) is a private, nonprofit, nonresidential, community-based distance-education graduate school offering a master of science in nursing degree and certificates in advanced practice specialties. The focused mission of the school is to provide a high-quality education that prepares nurses to become competent, entrepreneurial, ethical, and compassionate nurse-midwives and nurse practitioners who will provide primary care for women and families residing in all areas, with a focus on rural and medically underserved populations. The program is designed to offer greater flexibility in graduate education for mature, self-directed adult learners who prefer independent study or who are unable to relocate to existing programs that offer the nursing specialties provided in this program. It is a graduate program based on the concept of community-based distance learning, a "university without walls." One foundational concept of a community-based education program is that students learn best in their home environments. They do not leave the community they plan to serve in order to gain nurse midwifery or nurse practitioner education, and they use the resources of that community as part of their learning environment.

The school operates community-based programs that consist of four levels of instruction. All courses in Level I, II, and IV are offered year-round with the student able to start and finish a course on his or her own schedule. Level III requires a 2-week on-campus residency. The curriculum plan for each track can be viewed in the FSMFN online catalog at www.midwives.org/catalog.

All students come to the Hyden, Kentucky, campus for Frontier Bound, a 6-day intensive orientation to the school that includes introduction to all Level I courses by the faculty, meetings with advisors, computer and library instruction, and, most important, bonding with each other and the faculty and staff so that they will not feel isolated when they return home. Students return home to complete Web-based courses for Level I, the foundational courses for practice; and Level II, the foundational courses for management. Students interact with each other, faculty, staff, and alumni using the FSMFN Web portal system, named the Banyan Tree, for course work, social support, and scholarly inquiry into practice issues. The student returns to campus for Level III, a 2-week intensive skill training and verification experience. Level IV focuses on clinical practice and the course work that is best suited for learning while in practice. The clinical practice is done in a community-based clinical site that has been assessed by the Frontier faculty and deemed an appropriate site for learning. Students are guided in the clinical area by expert clinical faculty. Problem solving and developing independent decision-making are integral parts of the clinical practicum. They are seeing patients, making diagnostic and management decisions, and, if a midwifery student, assisting mothers during childbirth. Students have a minimum of 675 hours of clinical practice as part of their course of study.

After completing their clinical courses, including the preceptor's signing a Declaration of Safety, the student takes a comprehensive examination covering all course work. Passing the examination leads to graduation. Although the formal graduation ceremony occurs only once each year in October, a student graduates the day the faculty member verifies that the student has passed the comprehensive examination.

More than 1,070 nurse-midwives have graduated from this program, representing every state in the nation. In 2000, FSMFN began the Community-Based Family Nurse Practitioner Program (CFNP), making family nurse practitioner education available through community-based learning. As of fall 2004, 24 family nurse practitioners have also graduated from this program. The innovative, nonresidential, community-based program allows nurses to become advanced practitioners using their own communities as their classrooms.

During the 1990s, the school's focus was the implementation of the highly successful CNEP program for nurse midwives. The program was a certificate program with an option for completing a master of science in nursing degree through an affiliation agreement with the Frances Payne Bolton School of Nursing at Case Western Reserve University (FPBSON/CWRU). Students earned the MSN by completing nine credits for three courses that are offered several times a year in 1- and 2-week course intensives on the FPBSON/CWRU campus in Cleveland, Ohio. When the CFNP program was developed based on the CNEP model, the affiliation agreement was extended to include the CFNP students. For the nurse-midwifery students, completing the MSN was an option, depending on the requirements of the state where they lived, because in most states nurse-midwives could practice with a certificate. For the CFNP students, the MSN was mandatory in order to be eligible to sit for the national certification examination.

The FPBSON/CWRU affiliation was a wonderful asset to the program because FSMFN did not have institutional accreditation and could only offer certificate programs. As master's education for advanced practice nurses became the norm in the late 1980s and through the 1990s, this became an essential component of education for nurse-midwives as well as nurse practitioners. More than 80% of the CNEP students took advantage of this option and went to Cleveland to complete their MSN. The early CFNP graduates all completed their MSN through this affiliation. But as the geographical location of the students expanded to include all of the United States and seven foreign countries, the ability of students to go to Cleveland to complete intensive, on-campus courses declined. The FSMFN board of directors and administration recognized that this was becoming more and more of a barrier for students. Students and graduates asked, "Why can't we do the MSN courses at Frontier?"

STRATEGIC PLANNING GOALS FOR MSN PROGRAM

In 1999, the FSMFN board of directors, administration, and faculty began strategic planning sessions with a focus on the development of a master of science in nursing program with tracks in nurse-midwifery and family nurse practitioner education. There was much work to be done. The goal was to provide a superior education using distance technologies, allowing students to remain in their home communities as much as possible during their education. Twelve strategic planning goals with a 5-year timeline were developed and approved by the board of directors. The rest of this chapter outlines those objectives and the progress made.

Design, Implement, Evaluate, and Improve the Revised Graduate Curriculum

Recognizing that the first step in the path toward full accreditation must be to develop the MSN curriculum, a major revision to the curriculum was planned and completed in the year 2000. This was necessary to assure that the curriculum for the planned master of science in nursing (MSN) degree met all of the criteria established for this degree by the Southern Association of Colleges and Schools (SACS), the American Association of Colleges of Nursing (AACN), the American College of Nurse-Midwives (ACNM), the National Organization of Nurse Practitioner Faculty (NONPF), the National League for Nursing Accrediting Commission, and the National Certification Corporation for the Obstetric, Gynecologic, and Neonatal Nursing Specialties (NCC). An eminently qualified nurse educator, Carol Panicucci, PhD, FNP, was hired and appointed as coordinator of graduate curriculum. Her charge was to lead the curriculum revision, assuring that all competencies were met while avoiding duplications. The process included a series of conference calls culminating in an on-campus 4-day retreat of the entire faculty. Additions to the curriculum included strengthening the women's health content for the Community-Based Family Nurse Practitioner Program (CFNP) and strengthening the primary care content for the Community-Based Nurse

Midwifery Education Program (CNEP). Two new courses were added to meet the needs of the MSN students for a foundation in theories related to primary care and research. The new curriculum was implemented in the fall of 2000.

The curriculum committee developed and implemented an annual evaluation process that includes course analysis and review of graduate outcomes, as well as biannual peer-evaluation of each course. Course content is determined by the competencies defined by the professional organizations and by the mission of the FSMFN. In addition, the FSMFN is committed to teaching the principles of effective business management, with the goal that practitioners will have the skills to open and operate their own practices. As each course is revised, the faculty member reviews the curriculum map, the student course evaluations, peer reviewer comments, and national exam results and uses these data to plan the course revision. The depth of the revision is based on the need that is revealed through this data analysis. When the revision is completed, it is sent to the curriculum committee. There, it is reviewed by the coordinator of graduate education and two assigned faculty peer reviewers. The course is made available to all course coordinators, allowing others to assist the faculty member in improving the course. Comments from these reviews are used by the course coordinator to complete the course revision. After the course obtains curriculum committee approval, it is sent to the multimedia team who works with the course coordinator to add edits and any new technology pieces that might be requested by the course coordinator. The course is then placed on the FSMFN Web site. To evaluate the curriculum as a whole, the FSMFN uses a systematic plan to evaluate continuously the terminal MSN and specialty track objectives through 1-year and 5-year graduate and employer surveys, certification results, and comprehensive examination results.

Achieve Licensure and Accreditation From Appropriate Organizations

Licensure

In 2000, the FSMFN applied to the Kentucky Council on Postsecondary Education to include the master of science in nursing degree in the areas of nurse-midwifery and family nurse practitioner with our license. Approval was received on October 17, 2000.

Institutional Accreditation

In 2000, FSMFN actively began the process to achieve institutional accreditation through the Southern Association of Colleges and Schools

(SACS). School administrators first attended a SACS orientation session in January 1999 and attended a second session in January 2000. The orientation made it apparent that there was much work to do in terms of the way the school was organized, the implementation of the new graduate curriculum, and the development of an effective institutional effectiveness process.

In order to meet the criteria laid out by SACS, the school organization had to be restructured. The SACS criteria require that the school have a chief executive officer whose primary responsibility is to the institution and who is not the presiding officer of the board. The FSMFN is one of five not-for-profit subsidiary corporations of the Frontier Nursing Service. The five corporations include a critical access hospital, four rural health clinics, the school, the historic real estate, and the FNS Foundation. In 2000, the dean, who reported to the president of the school, led FSMFN. The president of the school was also the president of all five FNS corporations. The school did meet the requirement of having a separate board of directors. In 2001, Susan Stone, DNSc, CNM, was appointed president and dean of the school. The president and dean report directly to the FSMFN board of directors. Two department chairpersons were also appointed: Julie Marfell, ND, FNP, as the chair of Family Nursing, and Suzan Ulrich, DPh, CNM, as chair of Midwifery and Women's Health. The reorganization allowed the school to operate efficiently with a relatively flat hierarchy, which allows decisions to be made and plans to move forward with very little administrative delay (see Figure 10.1).

In June 2001, the school submitted the first application for candidacy to SACS. Feedback led to the separation of the school from the FNS, Inc. administrative structure. In fall 2001, a second application was submitted with feedback requiring expansion of the physical library facilities. In February 2002, a third application was submitted. At the SACS annual meeting in December 2002, the school was notified that it had been approved for a candidacy site visit. The school hosted six site visitors from SACS at the school in March, 2003. In June 2003, the FSMFN received approval as a candidate for accreditation with the Commission of Colleges of the Southern Association of Colleges and Schools. Members of the school administrative team met with the SACS liaison in July 2003 in Atlanta, Georgia, to continue the process to full accreditation. A leadership team was appointed and began the process of writing the SACS compliance document, which was submitted in May 2004. In July 2004, the accreditation site visit was completed with a team of six site visitors inspecting all aspects of the school for compliance. The final report was very positive and offered no recommendations to the school. The decision regarding full accreditation was made at the annual SACS/ COC Commission Meeting in December 2004.

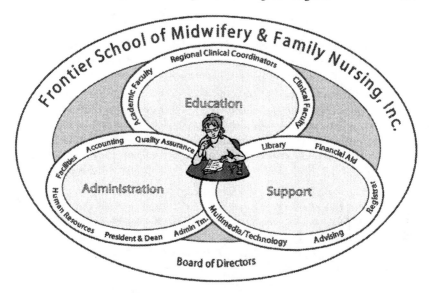

FIGURE 10.1   FSMFN organizational structure.

Program Accreditation

Knowing that the school would need the approval of the American College of Nurse-Midwives Division of Accreditation (ACNM/DOA) to offer the MSN program to the CNEP students, a change of status was requested in February 2002. A change of status from a certificate program to a master of science in nursing program was approved in February of 2002.

Accreditation through the National League for Nursing Accreditation Commission (NLNAC) was also pursued. This was necessary to operate the CFNP track and to provide overall validity to the MSN program. Because a scheduled review from the ACNM/DOA was planned in fall 2004, a coordinated site visit with both NLNAC and ACNM/DOA participating site visitors was completed in October 2004. The program received full accreditation status by both ACNM/DOA and NLNAC in February of 2005.

Develop, Evaluate, and Improve Library Resources

Improvement of the quality of library services in order to meet the needs of the graduate-level program was a necessary goal. In the earlier days of the program, students were sent course packs with all of their required articles included. They could order articles through the FSMFN library but access was very limited. Most used their local libraries either in the college of nursing where they had done their undergraduate education or through their employers, many of which were hospitals with good library resources. Although this had served the students fairly well, it was not a reliable method, and the faculty was committed to providing adequate library services and improving the information literacy skills of students in the graduate program. To start the improvement process, a fully qualified half-time librarian was hired. In addition, FSMFN contracted with the University of Kentucky Medical Library to provide expert consultation and support. Strategic planning goals were developed for the library, which guided the development of a comprehensive online library that is continuously available to faculty and students on-site and off-site. The on-site physical collection focuses on primary care and midwifery resources that students need only when on campus. The new library provides for adequate physical space and includes a fully equipped computer lab that students use during their on-site sessions. With full support from the FSMFN board of directors, a large building on campus called Aunt Hattie's Barn was renovated. The library and a large, well-equipped computer lab moved into this space in 2003. A dedicated high-speed T1 line and wireless access for the campus were added. This speeds up access to library resources both when on campus and when at home. Wireless access cards are made available to on-site students, allowing access to courses, the communication system, and library services.

Today the school has a full-time qualified librarian and offers a comprehensive online library focused on primary care nursing and midwifery that is available to faculty and students anyplace and anytime. A well-organized library Web site facilitates the use of the library. An online tutorial and an introduction to library services at Frontier Bound assists the students in becoming information literate. The fully equipped physical library includes two computer access stations and 10 computer access stations in the computer lab on the second floor. A very active library committee includes the librarian, faculty, students, and a Web designer, who continuously evaluate the current library resources to meet the needs of the FSMFN community.

Develop, Evaluate, and Improve the Use of Technology to Support Teaching and Learning

In 2000, all courses were developed in paper format and placed into paper modules and mailed to students. Although e-mail and forums were used extensively, the courses themselves were not available on the Web. The goal was to develop all courses in a format that facilitated Web-based delivery from a user-friendly Web site. The design team was recruited; Heather East, BA, was appointed multimedia director; and the process began.

Today all courses are delivered through a central Web portal. In addition, these are supported by a rich interactive communication system. Every course has its own discussion forum. Faculty members use many different modalities in their teaching, including verbal course introductions, online chats, PowerPoint presentations, mini tests, and games. Most assignments are received through e-mail attachments, allowing efficient turnaround time to students. News, activities, calendars, and group activities are communicated electronically. The Web site communication system has become a successful online community that exchanges more than 2,000 messages per day. All of these modalities are available to students, faculty, and staff 24 hours a day, 7 days a week. (The public site can be accessed at www.midwives.org.) The Web portal is password protected and available only to members of the FSMFN community.

Increase Financial Resources

The school is primarily funded through tuition and fees. Students pay $350/credit hour if full-time and $375 credit/hour if part-time. The program credits are as follows:

> MSN—CNEP track: 66 credits
>
> CNEP certificate: 60 credits
>
> MSN—CFNP track: 57 credits
>
> CFNP post-master's certificate: 51 credits

Eighteen percent of all school expenses are funded through the Frontier Nursing Service Foundation. A very effective fund-raising campaign held in the 1980s provided a sizable fund designated for the school, called the Nurse Education Enrichment Drive (NEED), which continues to provide substantial support. This allows the school to maintain an affordable tuition rate. The FNS Foundation also manages 10 different scholarship funds, which provide annual scholarships for students who meet the criteria and apply. In addition, the school has received support from the HRSA Division of Nursing Nurse Traineeship Program for the past 10 years. Efforts are focused on continuing to build the NEED and scholarship funds. Plans are in place to hire a dedicated development officer to assist in these efforts.

Improve Student Retention

Attrition was identified as an area of concern in the year 2000. In 2001, the attrition rate hit an all-time high of 23%. The faculty and staff came together to develop an action plan to address this issue. Students participated in the planning. The student advisor role was completely reorganized. Students activated the Mi Amiga (my friend) student support system. Faculty were gradually transitioned from primarily part-time positions to primarily full-time positions, including responsibilities for student advising. This provided more time to attend to the needs of students. A faculty "Mom" program was started where each student had a faculty "Mom" they would connect to during the on-site orientation. This was eventually replaced by having an assigned faculty advisor who had responsibility for a specialty track class of students. Each class has its own online forum and the faculty advisor monitors and participates in the forum. A part-time option was implemented that allows the students to complete the program in 3 years instead of 2. Above all, the faculty and staff worked very hard to develop a culture of caring. The message that faculty, administration, and support staff are there to assist the students to be successful is pervasive. Students are encouraged to call anytime they feel discouraged or have a problem. The result was outstanding: As shown in Figure 10.2, the attrition rate fell rapidly. The attrition rate for 2003 and 2004 was 6%.

Establish a Research Agenda

Establishing a research agenda has been a slow process. It has been clear from the beginning that there would be a focus on institutional effectiveness, clinical issues, and educational issues. One necessary goal identified was to increase the number of doctorally prepared faculty members. (At the beginning of this process, there were none.) In 1999 one was hired, in 2000 two were hired, in 2001 two were hired, in 2002 one was hired, and in 2004 one more was hired. A faculty tuition assistance program was established. One faculty member started a doctoral program and finished in 2002. Five faculty members are currently enrolled in doctoral programs with two more planning enrollment in 2005. There are currently seven full-time and one part-time doctorally prepared faculty members. This faculty is now poised to do clinical research.

Develop Faculty Practice

The next goal was to establish a faculty practice; a place where the effectiveness of nurse practitioner and nurse-midwifery care could be

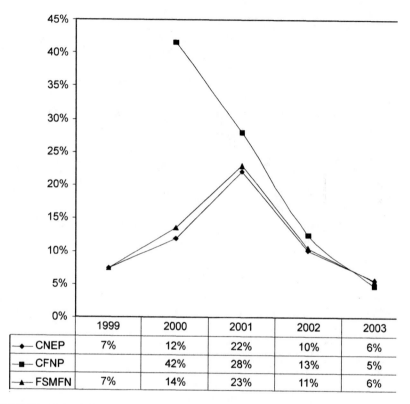

	1999	2000	2001	2002	2003
♦— CNEP	7%	12%	22%	10%	6%
■— CFNP		42%	28%	13%	5%
▲— FSMFN	7%	14%	23%	11%	6%

FIGURE 10.2   FSMFN attrition rates 1999–2003.

demonstrated. The obvious choice was the FNS rural health clinics. In 2002, FSMFN took over the management of the rural health clinics' clinical staff. Faculty members provide all clinical services. Any nurse practitioner or nurse-midwife recruited to work in the clinics became an employee of the school and a member of the faculty practice. This provided the school with clinical faculty and provided Frontier Nursing Healthcare (FNH) with needed clinicians. It also established an optimum place to conduct clinical research on the effectiveness of nurse practitioner and nurse-midwifery care. In 2003, FSMFN Chair of Family Nursing Julie Marfell was appointed as the executive director of the Frontier Nursing Healthcare rural health clinics. A complete evaluation of electronic medical records systems resulted in the purchase of a new system. The electronic system provides medical record management, a billing system, and data collection. This data collection function will provide health process and outcome data.

Integration of Practice and Research

The combined actions of increasing the number of doctorate-prepared faculty, establishing a clinical practice environment, and implementing a system that will track data provides a solid base to move forward and do clinical research. Faculty continue to move forward toward the goal of establishing a program of research at FSMFN. In 2004, after lengthy discussions in the faculty forum, the faculty voted on a definition of scholarship and how they will implement this definition as part of their faculty responsibilities. The adoption of this statement is part of the process that this faculty is engaged in to develop their scholarly identity. The agreed upon scholarly focus is evaluative research related to advanced nursing practice:

FSMFN Statement of Scholarship

Scholarship at the Frontier School of Midwifery and Family Nursing (FSMFN) is defined as those activities that systematically advance the teaching, research, and practice of midwifery, family nursing and women's health care through rigorous inquiry.

We concur with Boyer's (1990) assertion that:

"Theory leads to practice. But practice also leads to theory. And teaching at its best shapes both research and practice. Surely scholarship means engaging in original research. But the work of the scholar also means stepping back from one's investigation, looking for connections, building bridges between theory and practice and communicating one's knowledge effectively to students."

At FSMFN the scholarship of teaching, research and practice are all equally valued. We believe that the three form a continuum that strengthens each other.

For our work to be considered scholarly it must meet the following criteria as cited by Boyer (1990).

1. Clear goal
2. Adequate preparation (investigation of what is known)
3. Appropriate method (disciplined and systematic)
4. Significant contribution
5. Effective presentation
6. Reflective critique

We continue to explore a broad definition of the term "scholarly work" that includes a wide variety of activities that contribute to the advancement of knowledge. We are committed to using these six criteria to define and evaluate our scholarly work. (FSMFN Faculty Handbook, 2004)

Continue New Program Development

This goal included development and implementation of the Women's Health Nurse Practitioner Program and the combined CNM-FNP program of study. The FSMFN sought to establish both a Women's Health Nurse Practitioner Program (WHNP) track in the MSN program and a certificate program. Licensure from the Kentucky Council on Postsecondary Education to operate a WHNP program was received in 2001. After a review of the program, approval was obtained from the National Certification Corporation (NCC) for CNEP graduates to add one more clinical course to their curriculum to be eligible to sit for the national WHNP examination. Nine students graduated with a WHNP certificate in 2003. Although a curriculum for a separate WHNP track was developed, it was decided it would be best to implement such a program after FSMFN receives full accreditation from SACS and NLNAC. It is important that nurse practitioners graduate from a fully accredited program. This goal will move forward to 2005.

A program plan was developed whereby students seeking certification as both a nurse-midwife and family nurse practitioner could follow an efficient and effective path to meet their goals. The program plan allows students to do each program consecutively without duplication of course work. Upon graduation they are eligible to sit for both CNM and FNP national certification exams. Two students have completed this program and three more are currently enrolled.

Increase Offerings in Continuing Education

Using the revised and updated curriculum, several courses needed by nurse-midwives and nurse practitioners are offered as nonmatriculated courses to practitioners who need to update their knowledge base. These courses include pharmacology, physical assessment, and primary care I. All are Web-based courses that do not require any on-campus sessions. An average of seven preceptors or alumni take these courses each year. Two courses designed to educate clinical preceptors in teaching skills were developed in 2004. One is a modular-based book. The other is

delivered via CD-ROM. Both courses are distributed to all current preceptors. One focus in 2005 will be the evaluation of these programs.

Develop a Comprehensive Facilities Management Plan

In each of the past three years, the facilities management plan has been
revised and improved. The plan started with an assessment of the FSMFN
facilities and what was needed to provide a safe and satisfying environment for students, faculty, and staff. The maintenance plan maps out 10
years of planned improvements of all campus facilities. Assessments of
facilities are included in all student on-site evaluations. Many new improvements related to safety, security, and technology were added to all
campus facilities. The school maintains the historic appearance of all
the campus buildings while at the same time implementing a wireless,
technologically advanced environment.

Develop, Implement, Evaluate, and Improve a Comprehensive Plan for Institutional Effectiveness

The FSMFN administration, faculty, and staff have worked diligently to
improve the process of institutional effectiveness during the past 4 years.
Institutional effectiveness has become a major goal, affecting all school
activities. Administrators and faculty regularly attend the annual meeting
of the Southern Association of Colleges and Schools (SACS). Many excellent sessions are offered regarding the principles and implementation of
an effective educational plan that includes circular goal setting, planning,
and evaluation. The process has become ingrained.

The first activity was to develop a clear mission statement. Faculty,
staff, and FSMFN board members participated in this process. The
FSMFN board of directors adopted the mission statement in 2002. Every
5 years the board of directors, with the participation of the administration
and faculty develops 5-year objectives that are directly related to the
mission statement. At the beginning of each calendar year, using input
from the FSMFN community, an annual strategic plan is developed. In
this plan, goals and objectives for the coming year are defined. It is
essential that goals be stated in measurable terms, that they are evaluated,
and that the information gained from analysis of the information be used
to plan future programs and improvements. In the year 2003, a consultant
was hired to assist in the development of the comprehensive plan for
institutional effectiveness. The consultant reviewed the planning process
and then came to the FSMFN annual fall faculty meeting where he pre-

sented to the faculty and staff regarding the meaning of institutional effectiveness. With his assistance, the faculty brainstormed strengths and limitations in this area. He pointed out that although evaluations are done (for example, course evaluations, student satisfaction surveys, faculty satisfaction surveys, board of director evaluations, Frontier Bound evaluations) there was not always documented evidence that the results are used to improve processes. Oral history is insufficient; documented use of evaluation tools is required. The result was a new format for the planning and evaluation process. Figure 10.3 represents the FSMFN Planning and Evaluation Process.

The result is a very comprehensive institutional effectiveness plan. Goals are carefully devised, and measurable objectives are in place for every goal. Evaluation tools for each course and every activity are carefully constructed and implemented. Systems are in place that allow all constituents to access evaluation results to be used in further planning. A quality enhancement section of the FSMFN portal has been developed that collates all school evaluations and outcomes. For example, instructors can access their course evaluation results at any time. This facilitates use in further course development.

A graduate survey is completed every January. All graduates, and their employers, who are 1 year out and 5 years out are asked to fill out the survey. The data are placed on the Web site and used by the faculty to identify the strengths and weaknesses of the program. Attending SACS conferences, using consultants, implementing structured processes, and paying close attention to the process and the outcomes all have contributed to steady improvement in this area. The evaluation process has resulted in improved quality across the board. The school has always evaluated its processes and outcomes but the systematic method of staying true to the mission and objectives has now become embedded in the culture, providing a continuous commitment to the cyclical evaluation process.

OUTCOMES

Students and Graduates

In 2003, FSMFN graduated the first class of MSN students. Seventeen students graduated on October 18 with a master of science in nursing degree. There are currently 120 students enrolled in the MSN program. During the calendar year of 2003, 268 students attended the school. This included 227 in the nurse midwifery track and 41 in the family nurse

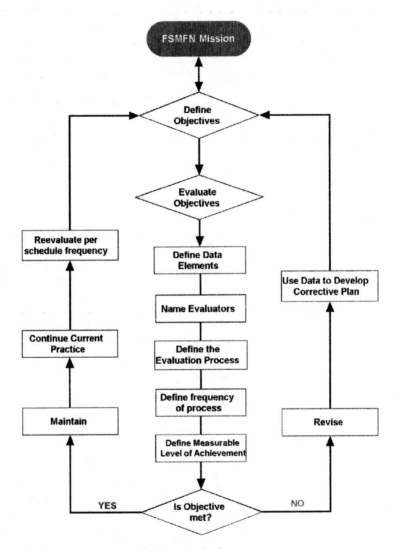

FIGURE 10.3 FSMFN evaluation method.

practitioner track. Nine enrolled in the Women's Health Nurse Practitioner completion option. Three are currently enrolled in a dual program plan with intentions of completing both the nurse-midwifery and the family nurse practitioner tracks. Twelve of the CNEP students participated in the Women's Health Nurse Practitioner completion option. The average age of students is 39 years old. Of the 268 students, 246 were Caucasian, 15 were African American, two were Hispanic, one was Asian, three were American Indians, and one was Iranian. The students represented every single state in the Union by their geographical place of residence. There were 262 women and 6 men enrolled. A total of 89 new students attended the Frontier Bound orientation sessions. This represents a 7% increase in enrollment compared to 2002. A total of 107 students participated in the clinical portion of their education, using 149 clinical sites. Students attending the Level III on-site, 2-week sessions totaled 61. A total of 200 or 75% of students participated in the Federal Financial Aid Program.

Faculty

FSMFN has a dedicated complement of 32 teachers, administrators, and librarians. Of this number, 16 are full-time, and 16 are part-time. All but two of the part-time faculty are regional clinical coordinators (RCCs). RCCs are clinical faculty whose main priority is to provide advising services to students and clinical faculty during the clinical portion of the students' education. This includes making preclinical site visits to evaluate the suitability of a site and clinical site visits when a student is at the site. RCCs are assigned to cover a specific geographic region. All faculty have a minimum of a master's degree, with seven having doctoral preparation. All are certified in their area of specialty, with five holding certification as both nurse-midwives and family nurse practitioners. Six faculty members are currently pursuing doctorates.

Support Staff

The FSMFN staff includes a group of devoted professionals intent on providing excellent support services to the students. The staff includes the registrar, the financial aid officer, and the quality assurance coordinator (QAC). The QAC handles all arrangements for clinical site placement. This includes working with the clinical sites to arrange the site visits and establish contracts before any student is placed at the site. There is also a four-member multimedia team that builds all the courses, manages the technology infrastructure, and provides technical support to students, faculty, and staff.

Graduation Report

A total of 53 students completed the CNEP in 2003. Of the 53 CNEP graduates, 19 also received a master of science in nursing degree. Additionally, nine of the CNEP graduates completed the added course work to obtain a Women's Health Nurse Practitioner certificate. A total of eight students graduated from the CFNP. Of the eight CFNP graduates, five also received a master of science in nursing degree. One student completed both the CNEP and CFNP.

Evaluation Results

Results on the national certification exam are one indicator of the quality of the curriculum and the program. The 2003 results for the ACNM Certifying Corporation (ACC) examination show that CNEP graduates had a 92% first-time pass rate compared to a 76.2% national first-time pass rate. All CFNP graduates have passed the national certifying exam the first time. Results of the graduate survey completed in January 2004 (see Table 10.1) reveal that CNEP graduates are employed in their specialty and are serving underserved clients. Some are also running their own practices. There were five graduate surveys sent out for the CFNP track. Two were returned, which does not allow for any grouped data analysis.

CONCLUSION

The Frontier School of Midwifery and Family Nursing engaged in a purposeful plan to convert its distance-education certificate programs to an online master of science in nursing degree offering for nurse-midwives and nurse practitioners. The result is a high-quality program that provides excellent educational opportunities at the graduate level for nurses who desire to further their education but cannot leave their home communities or who need to study on their own schedules.

TABLE 10.1   Employment Data from FSMFN 2004 Graduate Survey

	1-Year Graduates	5-Year Graduates
Employed as CNM	89%	87%
Working in Underserved Areas	34%	41%
Serving Medicaid Clients	86%	96%
Running Their Own Practice	17%	16%

REFERENCES

Stone, S., Ernst, E., & Shaffer, S. (2000). Distance education at the Frontier School of Midwifery and Family Nursing: From midwives on horseback to midwives on the World Wide Web. In J. Novotny (Ed.), *Distance education in nursing* (pp. 180–198). New York: Springer.

FSMFN (2004). Frontier School of Midwifery and Family Nursing Faculty Handbook, Hyden, KY.

CHAPTER 11

Supervising RN Students in an RN to MSN Program: Vanderbilt University School of Nursing

Carolyn J. Bess

The characteristics of registered nurse (RN) students that necessitate distance education approaches include social role commitments and adult learner attributes. RNs are working adults who fulfill family roles, such as spouse and parent (Gomez, Ehrenberger, Murray, & King, 1998). RNs have identified the need for flexibility in scheduling and location of educational programs (Krawczyk, 1997). Distinctive adult learner characteristics that support the use of distance learning as an educational methodology include (a) desires independence, (b) exhibits self-motivation, (c) values relevancy of new knowledge and skill, and (d) responds positively to active learning. Distance learning provides an environment to foster independence and autonomy that is desired by the adult learner (Gomez et al., 1998; Herrin, 2001). Self-directed learning by identification of one's own learning needs and objectives is supported by distance learning methodology (Koeckeritz, Malkiewicz, & Henderson, 2002). In many distance learning offerings, the facilitation of collaborative learning events is evident. The participants create their own content (Cragg, 1994). The adult learner responds best when new knowledge and skills are associated with prior learning. Application of RNs' problem-solving skills to new knowledge and skills is an effective reinforcer of learning. The distance learning process promotes an active learner (Ryan, Carlton, & Ali, 2004; Sternberger, 2002).

Distance education programs have been reported to increase RN student enrollment in BSN programs (Gomez et al., 1998). As the trend to offer distance learning courses at institutions of higher education escalates, a paradigm shift is occurring that supports the use of the Internet for content delivery and processing (Ryan et al., 2004; Sternberger, 2002).

With this higher education paradigm shift in mind, the faculty of a nontraditional graduate nursing program redesigned the educational methodology for RN students. The RN student (admitted after completing 78 hours of prerequisite course work) was expected to meet objectives equivalent to a BSN program at the end of two semesters of full-time study. The purpose of redesigning the traditional instructional methodology was to increase RN student enrollment while maintaining the educational quality and rigor of the program. The goal was to weave and blend traditional and nontraditional approaches to increase flexibility related to time and location of the educational offerings, producing a modified distance learning component of the RN to master of science in nursing (MSN) program. The synchronous or face-to-face interaction between teachers and students was altered by scheduling 4-day or 5-day block classes approximately three to four times during a traditional 14-week semester. A variety of asynchronous formats were used. These formats included compact discs (CDs) with combinations of videotaped lectures, voice-over PowerPoint (VOPP) and voice-over psychomotor skills demonstrations, e-mail, online conferencing, and student-selected, faculty-approved preceptors or agencies located at the student's location.

INTEGRATED SYNCHRONOUS AND ASYNCHRONOUS INSTRUCTIONAL DESIGN

In the first semester, full-time RN students were expected to complete five required courses for a total of 14 semester credit hours. The one clinical course this semester focused on basic health assessment content and skills. The didactic component was completed by use of CDs with VOPP and voice-over demonstrations of focused and head-to-toe examinations. Students were given a month to view the psychomotor CDs and practice before returning to campus for instructor-monitored lab practice and lab practical examinations and write-ups. Seventy clinical hours were spent with advanced practice nurses or physician preceptors who were selected by the student and approved by the faculty. The relationship between the student and preceptor provided opportunities for the students to experience professional practice socialization, which is clearly identified as a desired educational outcome of Web-based nursing courses (Billings, Connors, & Skiba, 2001; Bolan, 2003). E-mail and phone communication was used for addressing students' and preceptors' questions. The students were required to submit two complete history and physical write-ups on patients (due dates at midterm and end of semester). History and physical write-ups and instructor feedback comments were exchanged with faculty members electronically (fax or e-mail attachments) or through mail. During the semester, quizzes were administered per computer, covering content from VOPP and required readings. Midterm and final clinical performance evaluation feedback forms were submitted by fax or mail.

The second required course in the first semester fostered critical thinking, lifelong learning, and professional role development. This 3-hour didactic course used a block lecture format spread throughout the semester. Because of the focus of this course, the face-to-face, instructor-to-student contact allowed for professional socialization, role modeling, and mentoring that have been reported as deficient in distance learning methodologies (Billings et al., 2001; Milstead & Nelson, 1998). Use of a journal-writing learning activity focused on developing critical thinking abilities throughout the entire semester. The use of e-mail for faculty and student interaction and student-to-student interaction was encouraged. The importance of group projects such as student group issue presentations used in this course have been found to be difficult for geographically distant students, but were valuable in fostering student-to-student interaction (Cartwright & Menkens, 2002; MacIntosh, MacKay, Mallet-Boucher, & Wiggins, 2002). Evaluation strategies employed in this course were a role paper assignment, critical thinking journal activity, and oral presentation by a student group on an issue important to nursing practice.

The third 2-hour didactic course taken during the first semester focused on population-based health care principles of prevention, health maintenance, and health promotion. The videotape of traditional lecture content (provided by CD and in real time on course site) was used for this course because more than 100 on-site students were enrolled in the same course. The videotaping required more precise planning related to course schedule, technician availability, and backup plans. Some audiovisual aides required more preparation time with this course. In addition, contingency plans were needed when CDs were not received as scheduled by mail. Online conferencing was used for questions and answers related to lecture content and home work papers. Separate student online chat rooms were available on request for student work group discussions. Evaluation methodology employed was multiple-choice quizzes administered by computer and multiple small paper assignments.

The required fourth 2-hour didactic course emphasized concepts and skills foundational to patient education. Concepts of learning, motivation, change, and continuous improvement were addressed to explore the processes necessary to change individual self-care behaviors. Face-to-face lectures and discussions based on case study were used to present the content. An experiential learning activity where the student identified a personal health behavior that needed changing was implemented. Using the processes taught in the course, students developed a personal improvement project and reported their results by a poster presentation at the last block course meeting. Students provided a summary of the improvement process, results obtained, and analysis of what they learned personally and professionally from this activity. Actively engaging the students in an experiential activity impacted all student learning styles (Bolan, 2003). Evaluation methods employed were case-study–based teaching plans and a personal improvement project.

The required fifth 4-hour didactic course examined the human experience of health and illness across the life span. The focus of the course was on complex and chronic health problems. A complete set of CDs containing videotaped traditional lecture content was provided to students in the first block. Reading assignments included textbooks and online journal articles. The instructor was available by e-mail to address questions about content. Examinations were administered by computer with 1-week windows in which students could take their examinations at any time of the day or night and receive immediate results after submission. After closing of each examination, the student could review their test, receiving the rationale for the correct answer. Evaluation methodology employed was four multiple-choice, computer-administered examinations.

The second semester consisted of five required courses. The clinical course required 105 hours of clinical practice with a focus on the family in the community. Through didactic content and community practice, this course emphasized epidemiologic and nursing processes to support family and community health. Clinical hours were spent at self-selected faculty-approved agencies located in the student's community (e.g., hospices and family shelters). Family analyses and community assessments were required. A written community-focused proposal and project were completed. E-mail communication for questions and answers and project feedback and approval were instituted. A midterm and final clinical performance evaluation feedback form was submitted by fax or mail by the student's agency preceptor.

A 2-hour seminar class addressed selected topics foundational to the students' practice role. This course met face to face for 1 to 2 hours, three times during the semester. The intent was to continue the professional role socialization process begun the previous semester and to continue to facilitate role modeling and mentoring. The remainder of the course activities were online conferencing with faculty and student leadership and participation. Online conference setups included forums for course announcements, questions and answers, and five topic areas. Faculty-led forum topics were mentoring, Patricia Benner's model, collaborative practice model, and credentialing/certification process. Student-led forum topics were ethical issues related to specific populations (e.g., dying patients and premature or deformed infants).

Online chat rooms were available to each student leadership group to allow for discussion and planning for student-led forums. Online student responses were evaluated as to quantity and quality. The frequency of interactions was recorded without regard to quality. Quantity and quality was evaluated overall using the criteria in Table 11.1. The quality of student contributions was evaluated for each of the forums. Numerical scores representing quantity and quality were assigned for each student's participation in the forum. Quantity was represented by a simple count of postings. Quality was represented by $A = 4$; $B = 3$; $C = 2$; $F = 0–1$ based on the overall criteria. Increased frequency and quality of student interactions were found with online conferencing. This characteristic of online conferencing has also been identified by Ryan et al. (2004).

Students were expected to carry out leadership forum responsibilities. Groups composed of three students were assigned leadership responsibilities (see Table 11.2). Each student was evaluated on his or her individual leadership contributions to their forum in the areas of organization, completeness, relevancy, evidence-based interactions, and communication style. An additional evaluation strategy employed was annotated bibliographies focusing on forum topics submitted by e-mail attachments by all students.

The third and fourth required courses of the second semester addressed health care systems and related issues. These two didactic courses used videotape of traditional lecture format. E-mail communication to answer questions was implemented. Multiple choice examinations were administered. Written projects were submitted by e-mail attachments related to content on micro issues (e.g., leadership, team building, communication, and managerial skills) and macro issues (e.g., managed care, informatics, outcomes management, and financial management).

TABLE 11.1   Conferencing Participation Criteria

Grade	Criteria
A	Participates in all forums by making relevant comments and posing knowledgeable questions in reaction to material posted. Posts conference comments once a week. Reads all the required readings as indicated by relevant interactions. Posts evidence-based comments. Maintains a professional manner in all interactions with participants.
B	Participates in all but one forum by making relevant comments and asking topic-centered general questions in reaction to materials posted. Posts conference comments once a week. Reads most of the required readings as indicated by staying on discussion topics when interacting. Maintains a professional manner in all interactions with participants.
C	Participates in all but two forums by making general comments and asking vague questions in reaction to material posted. Posts conference comments once a week. Reads some of the required readings as indicated by inability to consistently stay on discussion topics when interacting. Maintains a professional manner in all interactions with participants.
F	Participates in four or less forums by making general comments and asking vague questions in reaction to materials posted. Posts conference comments less than once a week. Reads required readings inconsistently as indicated by inability to interact meaningfully on discussion topics. Maintains a professional manner in most interactions.

The last required course of the second semester addressed nursing theory and research. This 3-hour didactic and seminar course used face-to-face lecture and discussion methods to explore the content. Content included knowledge development in nursing, theoretical and research foundations for knowledge development, practice theory, scholarly inquiry to address professional nursing practice problems, research utilization, and evidence-based practice. Evaluation strategies employed were examinations, papers, and presentations. The blending of a variety of synchronous and asynchronous instructional strategies has provided RN students with flexibility related to time and location of their education.

IMPLEMENTATION ISSUES

Changing instructional methodology required preplanning to coordinate administrative support services (Milstead & Nelson, 1998). Services such

TABLE 11.2   Online Conferencing Student Leadership Responsibilities

Student	Responsibilities
1	To set the stage for the conference, this student posts a provocative opening statement introducing the conference topic. In the same forum thread, the student provides the participants a list of the forum's student leadership. This opening statement and leadership list should be posted on the first day of the 2-week forum. In addition to the introduction responsibilities, this student posts a forum summary at the end, identifying the major points covered during the 2-week forum. This summary statement should include major questions posed, significant comments made, and relevant areas explored by the participants and leadership during the forum. Summary statements are posted in the appropriate thread on the last day of the forum.
2	This student posts the case study for the conference discussion. The case study may be original or taken from another cited source. The case study should represent an ethical dilemma. Questions for discussion of the case study and the case study should be posted on the first day of the 2-week forum.
3	This student moderates the discussion by commenting on the other students' contributions and pointing out key concepts and ideas relevant to the topic discussion. In order to fulfill these responsibilities, the student must log on to the conference site and interact with the forum participants at least every third day during the 2-week conference period. This interaction should prompt participants' discussion by asking relevant questions to expand the discussion.

as registration were handled by mail or telephone. The nursing registrar's willingness to be flexible and the established procedure of student notification of registration deadlines by e-mail were essential. Student advisement was accomplished by a combination of phone, e-mail, and face-to-face appointments during block time segments. Although multiple communication methods were chosen by individual students, the most satisfying approach noted by this writer was the practice of setting individual short appointments during the last block dates of the semester. These 15- to 20-minute appointments addressed the student's view of how her or his program of study was progressing.

Support services, such as student orientation to the university and school of nursing community, was a 3-day segment attached to the first block class days. In addition to the standard student orientation, the distance student needed additional assistance related to computer technology and accessing library resources electronically. Basic computer technical resource requirements provided by the school's computer technology specialists were mailed to students as soon as they preregistered. This information was provided even to prospective students on request. Ongoing computer technical support was provided by the director of the Instructional Media Center and technically competent assistants. Technology problems experienced by students were related to difficulty in installing and using hardware and software and encountering server downtime and busy peak user times. The students found the technical support responsive, but their ability to identify the nature of a problem and communicate it successfully to the technical staff was problematic. As reported in the literature, we found that provision for technology support system to help distance students when problems occur was an essential component of a distance learning program (Cragg, Humbert, & Doucette, 2004; Milstead & Nelson, 1998).

Library services have presented a challenge. Librarians schedule appointments for groups of students to learn search skills during the orientation days. Distance students used online library databases and on-campus library resources during block class segments. Students who were resourceful found additional library services available in their own communities. Textbook availability was an issue related to timing. A block class segment was usually scheduled within the first week of classes. Students purchased textbooks and class packs at that time. Assigning required readings for the first block segment was problematic. Students could not complete all the reading assignments before class. Providing access to textbooks by mail and publishing textbook requirements and reading assignments for students 1 month prior to the first block class were instituted. These administrative services are key to providing a supportive educational environment for the distance student. Preplanning and coordinating these services were essential to the program's success.

An equally important aspect of a distant education program is the time and support provided to faculty members participating in this modified instructional methodology. Implementing a blend of synchronous and asynchronous instructional strategies has advantages and disadvantages. A disadvantage of using multiple technology approaches is based on the unfamiliarity of faculty and students in the application of technology to the learning process. As Ryan et al. (2004) recommended, we used a team effort to address this issue. The faculty members had computer technology specialists available for consultation, a multimedia production specialist was contracted for videotaping components, and faculty colleagues with a special interest in distributed learning were available to help plan online conferencing activities.

Advantages and disadvantages of the faculty role changes required were numerous. Faculty liked the increased flexibility of time scheduling but found the block class format a challenge to organize multiple learning activities to stimulate and motivate the learner. Faculty and students both liked the increased accessibility of faculty. E-mail and online conferences provided the capability to readily access faculty. As identified by Morris, Buck-Rolland, and Gagne (2002) and Ryan et al. (2004), there was an increase in faculty workload. More time was required with needed preplanning activities and team coordination. Faculty members needed to be involved in and informed of technology problems that adversely affected planned learning activities. If the server was down and the students did not post their assignments on time, then the faculty member needed to know. Maintaining alertness to actual and potential electronic problems that might affect the learning event was a new skill for many faculty. The support and counseling by other more experienced online educators were needed for faculty members participating in distance programs (Ryan et al., 2004).

Additional faculty time was needed to write messages, in contrast to in-class verbal interactions. Interactions in class are limited by time, but e-mail and conference postings were not limited by time and in many instances were not limited in volume (pages). The increase in volume of communication and increase in multiple thoughts being expressed in one student interaction required extra faculty time to process communication and organize a response. Changes in interpersonal interactions included a lack of visual and nonverbal cues when online communication occurred. The faculty noted that this lack tended to make interactions more impersonal and less spontaneous. Milstead and Nelson (1998) identified faculty personality characteristics that seem to counteract this tendency. These attributes were flexibility, patience, and an ability to employ a humanist online conversational language style. The use of block classes helped to offset this impersonal tendency and loss of spontaneity.

Changes in volume, pattern, and style of faculty-to-student and student-to-faculty interactions changed the faculty role. As identified by Kozlowski (2002), faculty members surrender control to learners and move to a facilitator-of-learning role when using online conferencing. When using a blend of synchronous and asynchronous instructional strategies, faculty members had to be flexible risk takers.

As students adapted to a different learning environment, student role changes were identified. Using a variety of instructional methodologies required the learners to be flexible. Students in most instances were learning new computer skills. As with any distance learning format, there is an increased responsibility placed on the learner (Atack, 2003; Billings et al., 2001). Emotional and interpersonal issues play a part in the student's adjustment to the autonomous distance-learner role. Students struggled with the sense of isolation that can occur with distance learning while the faculty used strategies to increase the learners' feeling of connectiveness (Billings et al., 2001; MacIntosh et al., 2002). Students had an increased need to develop and use their local resources, such as preceptors and agencies. Different types of demands are made on students' personal support systems, such as family, friends, employers, and fellow students. Students' written and verbal communication skills were challenged by distance methodologies. Communications were expected to be concise and condensed, organized, relevant, and evidence-based. Individual personalities and interpersonal dynamics impacted the quality of communications whether synchronous or asynchronous.

As with any group of students, variations in learning styles were expected. Providing a variety of instructional methodologies appeared to address this area of faculty concerns. This major concern was that using online conferencing and written assignments alone would be relying too heavily on the written word.

Another anticipated area of faculty concern in distance learning programs is providing opportunities for professional socialization (Billings et al., 2001; Milstead & Nelson, 1998). Online conferencing was set up to foster faculty-monitored group interaction. Chat rooms were made available to encourage student-to-student interactions. Planned synchronous class meetings were planned in block formats. A question-and-answer forum and e-mail both were monitored closely by course faculty members.

The clinical experience environment, when established by a distance, added to the students' responsibilities. The distanced students were expected to initiate setting up a preceptor or agency about 2 to 3 months in advance of the beginning of the semester. The students were sent a copy of the preceptor role and student responsibilities for the clinical experience. Student performance criteria detailing the expected behaviors were communicated in writing. Each student talked with the faculty member in charge to discuss potential appropriate sites. The student was provided directions for approaching preceptors by the contract office. The student then contacted a preceptor or agency and discussed his or her interest in working with the preceptor or agency. If the preceptor or agency was interested, the student communicated that interest to the faculty in charge of the course. If the site selected by the student was approved, the faculty member would initiate the contract process. A separate contract office existed in the school to assure coordination of clinical sites and standardization of records. Faculty members were available by phone during all steps in this process, to answer questions from students and potential preceptors and expedite the process.

To ensure instructional quality of the distance program, faculty sought both formative and summative evaluations. Student group debriefings were held face-to-face in block class segments of each semester. Students were encouraged to communicate by e-mail any concerns or problems when they occurred throughout the semester. Online course and instructor evaluations were administered during a 1- to 2-week window of time at the end of each semester.

SUMMARY

The design and implementation of an RN to MSN program to allow for modified distance learning was described. Instructional strategies to blend synchronous and asynchronous formats were employed. Two semesters of the program were described including each course focus, educational methodology and evaluation strategies. Educational methodology implemented included traditional lecture and seminar classes, delivered in 4-day and 5-day block classes three to four times during a semester, and asynchronous formats including CDs with combinations of videotaped lectures, VOPP and voice-over psychomotor skills demonstrations, e-mail, online conferencing, and student-selected faculty approved preceptors or agencies. Major distance-learning implementation issues discussed were preplanning essentials, technology challenges, faculty role changes, student role changes, clinical experience environment, and evaluating instructional quality. The purpose of the RN to MSN program design was to increase RN student enrollment while maintaining the educational quality of the program.

REFERENCES

Attack, L. (2003). Becoming a Web-based learner: Registered nurses' experiences. *Journal of Advanced Nursing, 44,* 289–297.

Billings, D. M., Connors, H. R., & Skiba, D. J. (2001). Benchmarking best practices in Web-based nursing courses. *Advances in Nursing Science, 23*(3), 41–52.

Bolan, C. M. (2003). Incorporating the experiential learning theory into the instructional design of online courses. *Nurse Educator, 28*(1), 10–14.

Cartwright, J. C., & Menkens, R. (2002). Student perspectives on transitioning to new technologies for distance learning. *Computers Informatics Nursing, 20,* 143–149.

Cragg, C. E. (1994). Distance learning through computer conferences. *Nurse Educator, 19*(2), 10–14.

Cragg, C. E., Humbert, J., & Doucette, S. (2004). A toolbox of technical supports for nurses new to web learning. *Computers Informatics Nursing, 22*(1), 19–25.

Gomez, E. G., Ehrenberger, H., Murray, P. J., & King, C. R. (1998). The impact of the national information infrastructure on distance education and the changing role of the nurse. *Oncology Nursing Forum, 25*(10), 16–20.

Herrin, D. M. (2001). E-learning: Directions for nurses in executive practice. *Journal of Nursing Administration, 31*(1), 5–6.

Koeckeritz, J., Malkiewicz, J., & Henderson, A. (2002). The seven principles of good practice: Application for online education in nursing. *Nurse Educator, 27*, 283–287.

Kozlowski, D. (2002). Using online learning in a traditional face-to-face environment. *Computers in Nursing, 20*(1), 23–30.

Krawczyk, R. (1997). Returning to school: Ten considerations in choosing a BSN program. *Journal of Continuing Education in Nursing, 28*(1), 32–38.

MacIntosh, J., MacKay, E., Mallet-Boucher, M., & Wiggins, N. (2002). Discovering co-learning with students in distance education sites. *Nurse Educator, 27*, 182–186.

Milstead, J. A., & Nelson, R. (1998). Preparation for an online asynchronous university doctoral course: Lessons learned. *Computers in Nursing, 16*, 247–258.

Morris, N., Buck-Rolland, C., & Gagne, M. (2002). From bricks to bytes: Faculty and student perspectives of online graduate nursing courses. *Computers Informatics Nursing, 20*, 108–114.

Ryan, M., Carlton, K. H., & Ali, N. (2004). Reflections on the role of faculty in distance learning and changing pedagogies. *Nursing Education Perspectives, 25*(2), 73–80.

Sternberger, C. S. (2002). Embedding a pedagogical model in the design of an online course. *Nurse Educator, 27*, 170–173.

CHAPTER 12

Distance Education at the University of South Carolina College of Nursing

Kristen S. Montgomery, Judith W. Alexander, Tracy Bushee, Mary Ann Parsons, and Vera Polyakova-Norwood

Distance education in nursing began in 1972 with the University of Mississippi Nurse-Midwifery Educational Program and since then has had an increasing impact on nursing education. In the late 1990s, distance and online education experienced significant growth. According to the Education Department's National Center for Education Statistics, in the 2000–2001 academic year, enrollment in for-credit distance education courses grew to 2.9 million. The survey conducted in 2002 found that 90% of public 2-year institutions and 89% of 4-year colleges and universities offered courses to students at a distance (Kiernan, 2003). The primary reason public educational institutions embraced distance and online education was to improve access to educational opportunities for the public and to keep the price of education at a reasonable level (Kiernan, 2003).

During the last decade nursing has witnessed a technological explosion in health care, and there is no sign that advances in technology are likely to dissipate anytime soon. Advanced technology permeates nearly every aspect of our personal and professional lives. Distance education in nursing has improved access to higher education for many nurses and has substantially improved nurses' career opportunities and knowledge. Distance education is particularly critical in rural states like South Carolina, where nurses are widely dispersed and fewer graduate programs exist compared to other areas of the country.

HIGHER EDUCATION IN SOUTH CAROLINA

Compared to more densely populated areas, rural areas typically have fewer university-level higher-education programs because there are fewer students to fill them. In contrast to many major cities that may have multiple major universities, South Carolina has three major public institutions of higher learning that offer nursing baccalaureate and higher-degree programs: the University of South Carolina (USC) system, the Medical University of South Carolina (MUSC), and Clemson University (CU). These three universities are located centrally with satellite campuses, in the southern region, and in the upstate, respectively.

NURSING EDUCATION IN SOUTH CAROLINA

South Carolina has multiple nursing programs distributed across the state at various levels. Both technical preparation (LPN and ADN) and collegiate preparation (BSN) exist. In addition to basic preparations, graduate programs exist at USC, MUSC, and Clemson. USC offers master's and post-master's education in a variety of specialties, as do MUSC and Clemson. Both USC and MUSC offer PhD programs in nursing and USC also offers the doctor of nursing degree (ND).

DISTANCE EDUCATION AT UNIVERSITY
OF SOUTH CAROLINA

University of South Carolina (USC) has a long history of distance education, dating back to the 1930s when the College of Independent Studies started offering correspondence courses statewide. Currently, 13 USC colleges offer selected courses and degree programs to students at a distance in the fields of education, public health, nursing, library and information science, business administration, engineering, and journalism. The largest distance education unit at the University of South Carolina is the Department of Distance Education and Instructional Support (DEIS, 2004) located on the central campus in Columbia, SC. Each semester more than a hundred courses are offered to degree-seeking students in a variety of delivery formats, including digital satellite broadcast (one-way video, two-way audio), videoconferencing (two-way video and audio), videocassettes, CD-ROM, DVD, print, and online technologies.

Among various distance education technologies available at USC, digital satellite broadcast remains a popular choice. USC and South Carolina Educational Television (ETV) have a long history of cooperation in statewide delivery of instructional programs. Each semester more than 40 live televised courses originate from USC's seven studio classrooms located on the main campus. This delivery method enables instructors to reach learners off campus without spending a considerable amount of time and effort in course redesign and development (Bates, 1995). Live televised courses also allow updating the learning content with the most recent information each time the course is offered.

Another advantage of the live broadcast is that students are not required to have any special equipment. For students in isolated rural areas where a broadband connection to the Internet is not available, live satellite broadcast remains the only option for taking courses with required participation in class sessions or rapidly changing content. To make satellite-delivered courses accessible to students off the main campus, the University of South Carolina has developed a wide network of viewing sites throughout the state.

The synchronous nature of live satellite broadcast, however, makes it less convenient for students with family responsibilities or busy work schedules. Other challenges of this model of distance education are limitations of the presentational capabilities of television in involving students at distant sites in interactive activities (Bates, 1995). Although the USC classroom studios are equipped with a telephone talk-back system, engaging students at distant sites in meaningful learning activities alongside their peers in the studio classroom requires additional planning and constant effort from the instructor.

The majority of distance education courses at USC, however, use a mix of technologies, which allows for a variety of instructional methods and formats within a single course. Previous work indicates that using multiple teaching methods is more likely to result in student learning. Online learning, often described as a new paradigm for teaching and learning (Harasim, 2000; Harasim, Hiltz, Teles, & Turoff, 1995; Kearsley, 2000), is rapidly gaining momentum and challenging older forms of distance education. A survey of USC's distance education students conducted in the spring semester 2003 indicated that 25% of the students participated in online learning, which is a threefold increase from the previous year (Hogue, 2003). Because this trend is likely to continue, USC's Strategic and Assessment Plan for Distance and Distributed Learning calls for enhancing existing distance education programs with new modes of delivery (Hogue, 2003).

In 1999, upon recommendation from the faculty, USC purchased Blackboard, an enterprise course management system. This enables instructors to create online courses and course components without investing a significant effort in learning HTML code and editing. Despite sporadic technical problems, the use of Blackboard quickly spread across academic departments and today the majority of USC faculty use this system to post course materials and resources on the Web, conduct synchronous and asynchronous discussions, manage homework and assignments, and distribute grades.

Since the acquisition of Blackboard, the number of courses delivered totally or partially online has been growing steadily. Although the number of degree programs available from USC entirely online is still small, several academic units have expressed an interest in launching online degree and certificate programs in the near future.

DISTANCE EDUCATION IN THE COLLEGE OF NURSING

University of South Carolina College of Nursing offered its first distance education course via closed circuit television in the 1984 spring semester. Nursing 700, Theoretical and Conceptual Foundations for Nursing, a graduate course, was offered at the nine regional campuses and at 31 hospitals throughout the state. The course was televised live on Saturday mornings. Students used talk-back via telephone to communicate with the instructor and fellow students.

During the 10 years following the first distance education offering, the number of distance education courses offered by the College of Nursing (CON) grew to more than 22, and in 2004 the number of distance education courses offered per semester varied between 8 and 12. Courses were offered within the MSN program, in the RN-BSN completion program, and the PhD program. In 1994, the College of Nursing's new television complex was used for the first time. This complex, a multipurpose, 52-seat studio has a wide-screen projector that benefits students viewing at a distance because they are able to see images more clearly. A presenter-driven computer with state-of-the-art multimedia technology is available in the studio to conduct distance education courses. Faculty are able to create presentations that include text, sound, full-motion video, and animation.

Starting in 2000, the College of Nursing began to develop online courses to meet the needs of distant students. The first course of this type was an undergraduate (RN-BSN) course, Nursing 410, Nursing Research. This course was developed collaboratively among the three campuses of the USC system. Alexander, Polyakova-Norwood, Johnston, Christensen, and Loquist (2003) describe use of the distance education literature to develop and evaluate the course. From that beginning in online teaching, several other courses in the RN-BSN program and a PhD seminar course were offered, using the online format for distance education.

Currently, the bulk of distance education courses are offered at the graduate (master's and ND levels). In these courses, students who reside in Columbia attend class on campus, which is delivered to students at distance sites via satellite. Distance education sites use closed circuit technology/phone at a variety of sites throughout the state. Students are generally required to be on campus for the first class session and perhaps once more during the semester for in-class activities like presentations, exams, or other work. Faculty generally limit on-campus class time to no more than two classes to preserve the conveniences of distance education, because students may travel 150 miles or more (each way) to come to Columbia and may be taking more than one course per semester on different days. When the online format is used, faculty members also use some face-to-face contact and have students come to campus at least once over the course of the semester. Currently, CON is not offering any courses using a totally online format.

ROLE OF THE FACULTY

In order to teach using distance educational methods, nursing faculty must be proficient in the use of the technology. When the format used is that of satellite broadcast in a live format, Distance Education and Instructional Support (DEIS) at USC provides a technician who sets up the studio and runs the camera. However, faculty must be aware of the limitations on movement and the use of the touch screen to switch the visuals displayed on the screen for the students (e.g., computer display, overhead projector, or video from the camera). Additionally, faculty must recognize the impact of color and font size on the quality of material that is used in broadcast. The same general skills are needed for presenting class content during video conferencing sessions or for content that will be videotaped or video-streamed for later use. This differs from general classes in that it may be more difficult for students to see materials via video that are projected in the classroom.

If an online modality is used, faculty need familiarity with how to post content on the course management software. Faculty at USC decided to use the universal HTML format to post material on Web sites for online courses so that students could access any part of the course with a Web browser without loading specific software, such as Microsoft Word or Microsoft PowerPoint.

Additionally, as suggested by many distance education experts (Harasim et al., 1995; Haughey & Anderson, 1998; Kearsley, 2000; Palloff & Pratt, 1999), transition to the online environment necessitated changes in the faculty-student relationship. The delivery of most of the course content is primarily through didactic methods (e.g., posting of HTML "lecture" notes on Blackboard); however, some portions of the course should introduce students to more active learning through moderated class discussions and guided exploration of Web-based resources. The latter teaching strategy requires faculty to develop questions that stimulate discussion, assess student learning in nontraditional ways, and provide interactivity among faculty and learners (Moore, 1989; O'Neil, Fisher, & Newbold, 2004).

With any distance-education course delivery modality, faculty must create a social presence. Social presence is the degree to which a person perceives other people as real and the degree to which learners feel the presence of their instructors (Gunawardena & Zittle, 1997). Posting a brief biographical note or picture on Blackboard is one way to do this.

ADMINISTRATIVE SUPPORT
FOR DISTANCE EDUCATION

Administrative support is critical to the success of distance education delivery. Policy decisions including teaching loads, faculty development, campus facilities, and technological support must be made with faculty and staff input. The "buy-in" of faculty and staff will vary based on the change culture in the college and must be considered in the decision to move forward with distance education. When decisions are made to move forward with new teaching modalities, including distance education, adequate resources and support from administration are essential to success. Particularly in the beginning when new initiatives are being launched, faculty will need adequate time, resources, and support services to ensure students and the course are successful. The College of Nursing has a history of strong administrative support for distance education offerings, which facilitated the early initiation of offerings in 1984 and continues today as the college proceeds to meet the future educational needs of nurses and those wishing to pursue nursing in the state of South Carolina.

ROLE OF THE UNIVERSITY AND UNIVERSITY SUPPORT

As faculty commit to develop various technology-based approaches, they can benefit from guidance and support from instructional developers and instructional technology specialists. Bates (1995) suggested that "instructional designers can play an invaluable role in helping subject matter experts define the various teaching and learning needs of a course, and making sure they are assigned to the most appropriate media" (p. 114). The university provides a wide range of support services to faculty who teach students at a distance, including assistance with course materials development, computer graphics enhancement, and hardware and software training. Instructional developers conduct workshops and offer group and one-to-one consultations for teaching through various distance education technologies.

In addition to the current support provided to faculty and students by the university, a Teaching and Learning Center is planned for 2005. This center will significantly increase opportunities for USC faculty to learn and use best practices in using various instructional models, share their experiences with colleagues, engage in inquiry about the impact of technology on the educational process, and explore teaching and learning issues in higher education at large.

One of the factors affecting students' success in distance education environments is the availability and quality of technical support provided by the institution (Harasim et al., 1995; Moore & Kearsley, 1996; Palloff & Pratt, 1999). Technical support for students in live televised courses is provided by Distance Education and Instructional Support (DEIS), which maintains equipment on the main campus and at participating viewing sites statewide. If students miss a class session because of problems with equipment or satellite transmission or reception, DEIS will mail them VHS tapes of that class session or will provide a video-streamed version of the class on the Internet. The latter option works well for students who have broadband access to the Internet at home.

Technical support for students and faculty participating in online courses delivered entirely or partially through Blackboard is provided by Computer Services. The help desk staff can be reached on the phone between 8 a.m. and 5 p.m. After hours and on weekends, students can submit a request for help on the USC Web site. This arrangement, however, may be inadequate for online learners who often need to access their course materials when immediate assistance is not available. Providing adequate technical assistance for rapidly growing numbers of online learners remains a challenge for the university's information technology (IT) office.

Other support services for distance learners include delivery of course materials, proctoring exams at distant sites, and returning assignments. Student services coordinators are available to distance students at a toll-free number during the regular work hours. USC libraries provide remote access to a large collection of online publications and research databases. Advisement and tutoring of distance learners fall within the responsibility of the academic departments.

The role of the university in supporting distance education is also critical. At the University of South Carolina, distance education is a major initiative. The university supports a rather large department of DEIS that manages the bulk of responsibilities related to the delivery of distance education courses. One key component of DEIS that is extremely helpful to faculty and students alike is that each department, school, or college within the university is assigned a specific instructional developer from DEIS to handle distance education course management. If a question arises related to distance education services, the faculty, staff, and students know immediately whom to contact at DEIS, which saves time, money, and frustration. An orientation is provided to faculty who are new to the university and to those new to teaching by distance education methods. A very comprehensive handbook also facilitates timely information retrieval related to distance education matters. Faculty members receive a video-taped copy of each class. Students also have the opportunity to meet the DEIS coordinator for their department, school, or college during the first class period when a brief orientation is provided. DEIS sends students materials prior to the beginning of class, which includes information on procedures related to taking a distance education course, the syllabus, contact information, procedures for completing course work, and other course materials. Distribution of additional materials, PowerPoint slides, and most outside of class communication occurs through Blackboard and e-mail. Weekly journals and other assignments are also accomplished through Blackboard when desired by the faculty teaching the course. When technical problems arise, students may request that a videotaped copy of the lecture be delivered to their viewing site. Students can then arrange a convenient time with the site to view the portion of class that was missed. Students may only request a videotaped copy for technical difficulties in producing the broadcast (such as equipment failures and thunderstorms); requests for tapes because of absences such as illness or work conflicts are not honored.

Faculty have the option of having students come to class for testing or testing can be accomplished at certain distance education sites where proctors are available. The regional campuses in the USC system, as well as some other sites, offer this option. In addition, with course management software like Blackboard, students can complete various types of exams online, and in the case of multiple-choice questions can receive immediate feedback. Results are automatically entered into the Blackboard gradebook for the faculty. Blackboard can be set to limit the length of time in which students may take the exam once they are signed in (e.g., a 1-hour limit); limits can also be placed on the specific days the exam can be administered and during what hours one wishes to permit students to take the exam. Both of these time features limit the possibility of cheating.

RESOURCES NEEDED FOR DISTANCE EDUCATION

Faculty development was a critical component to the college's move to distance education technology. Faculty members received funding to develop their multimedia expertise at courses on and off campus. A seed grant from the South Carolina Commission on Higher Education (CHE) was instrumental in facilitating the first online course. Faculty involved in that collaborative course provided online instruction development sessions for other faculty. Additionally, all faculty have a Blackboard site for each course they teach, whether the course is offered in the traditional format or using distance education. However, the college always has viewed distance technology only as a different educational delivery modality, and has not reduced teaching loads or given extra credit to faculty who teach using this methodology.

ISSUES RELATED TO STUDENT PERSPECTIVES OF DISTANCE EDUCATION

Most distance-education graduate students are balancing multiple demands during school, including the rigors of course work, outside employment, family, and running a household. These demands are the realities faced by most students in nursing who enroll in distance education courses. Though we cannot teach differently to students based on their outside demands, the structure of their busy lives does warrant consideration.

For distance education to be effective, it is essential for faculty to change the way they traditionally teach in the classroom. Both faculty and students must become proficient with the technology available to maximize the experience. DeBourgh (2003) presents various strategies faculty may use to promote student satisfaction in distance-delivered courses. These include inviting student contact in a variety of modalities (e.g., e-mail, online discussion boards, face-to-face and virtual office hours), and the effective use of instructional technology (for example, providing an online tutorial at the start of the course to ensure that students are able to use available course materials effectively).

Learning via distance education is most effective when it is student-centered (Kennedy, 2002). Faculty are encouraged to focus on "educational distance" rather than physical distance. When faculty focus on physical distance, they focus more on geography. When the focus is educational distance, delivery and support mechanisms engage students in understanding the material and communicating with colleagues and faculty in a personalized and collaborative learning process (Kennedy, 2002).

When courses are taught via video or online, students are able to view course material at a time convenient to them. However, one of the most important considerations of videotaped courses is the currency of the information. Courses such as pharmacology are often out-of-date by the time a videotaped course is used in a second semester. Although faculty can always meet with students to clarify information, it is ideal if updated information is presented initially. However, often schools must meet the demand for pharmacology faculty via creative arrangements, because they may be difficult to recruit. We have addressed these limitations by using videotaped sessions in only a limited number of courses and retaping courses annually to maintain currency of content.

Viewing exams can be a challenge with distance education courses. Unlike the traditional classroom setting where students are given the opportunity to review tests and learn why they missed questions, this opportunity may be neglected using a distance education format. Time set aside either on campus or virtually might assist students to feel more comfortable with the examination process in distance education courses. Time can be used to review exams and to clarify material students may not have understood.

Blackboard, review sessions, and assembling course packets with articles and book chapters to supplement the learning experience are techniques faculty can use to augment student learning in distance education courses. Periodic conferences following class that focus on a specific topic can also be useful in providing students opportunities to interact with each other and to reinforce important concepts from the reading and clinical experiences.

For students, technological problems are often the most frustrating experience associated with distance education. Addressing these issues prior to the beginning of the course is ideal. Changing the delivery format (e.g., from videotape to Internet) too close to beginning the class or switching formats mid-semester is also problematic. Last-minute downloads of software and reading materials can be problematic for some students, and other students may not be able to access the materials prior to the start of class without adequate notice. Streamlined video and slides that do not work properly are also frustrating. Technical assistance needs to be readily available 24/7 to assist students with problems related to technology. As online learning opportunities increase, institutions will need to make this level of technical support available to increase the recruitment and retention of students in such courses (Alexander et al., 2003). USC has "live" help during normal work hours and an e-mail contact to address problems after hours.

"Warmer" types of media such as videoconferencing, online chat discussions, and hybrid courses with a mix of online and face-to-face activities are more likely to encourage participant interactions (Atack, 2003). Faculty should also assist students to become comfortable with the technology they will need to successfully participate in the course. As suggested by Harasim et al. (1995), the course template should include an orientation unit to prepare students taking the course. In addition to providing guidance on how to use the technology, a module should introduce students to self-directed learning and contain initial community-building activities. Even with experienced distance-education learners, an orientation module is helpful to get all participants to know each other and clarify expectations for the course. An effective online community must be nurtured by faculty who carefully develop and sequence interactive learning activities (Carr & Farley, 2003).

By addressing the various aspects of distance education discussed, faculty can integrate the critical components needed to ensure that course objectives are met successfully. As technology continues to improve, distance education will have an even stronger presence. Student evaluations of distance education are useful for improvement. At USC, distance education students complete the same course evaluation form online as other students do, using traditional delivery formats. This evaluation incorporates some questions related to the distance education format and technical difficulties.

CONCLUSION

College of Nursing faculty are committed to continuing the use of distance education formats for course delivery. These pedagogies meet the needs of our students in a time of nursing shortage and information explosion. Students who otherwise might not be able to advance their education are able to enroll in nursing courses and earn degrees. In 2004, 20 years after our first venture into distance education delivery, closed circuit television, VHS tapes, videoconferencing, teleconferencing, compressed video, and online courses are used to deliver courses, making the College of Nursing a leader in distance education on campus and across the nation.

REFERENCES

Alexander, J. W., Polyakova-Norwood, V., Johnston, L. W., Christensen, P., & Loqusit, R. S. (2003). Collaborative development and evaluations of an online nursing course. *Distance Education, 24*(1), 41–56.

Atack, L. (2003). Becoming a Web-based learner: Registered nurses' experiences. *Journal of Advanced Nursing, 44,* 289–297.

Bates, A. W. (1995). *Technology, open learning and distance education.* London: Rutledge.

Carr, K. C., & Farley, C. L. (2003). Redesigning courses for the World Wide Web. *Journal of Midwifery and Women's Health, 48,* 407–417.

DeBourgh, G. A. (2003). Predictors of student satisfaction in distance-delivered graduate nursing courses: What matters most? *Journal of Professional Nursing, 19,* 149–163.

Distance Education and Instructional Support (DEIS). (2004). *Organizational units.* Retrieved October 11, 2004, from http://www.sc.edu/deis/about_us/organizational_units.html

Gunawardena, C. N., & Zittle, F. (1997). Social presence as a predictor of satisfaction within a computer mediated environment. *American Journal of Distance Education, 11*(3), 8–25.

Harasim, L. (2000). Shift happens: Online education as a new paradigm in learning. *The Internet and Higher Education, 3*(1–2), 41–61.

Harasim, L., Hiltz, S. R., Teles, L., & Turoff, M. (1995). *Learning networks: A field guide for teaching and learning online.* Cambridge, MA: MIT Press.

Haughey, M., & Anderson, T. (1998). *Networked learning: The pedagogy of the Internet.* Montreal, Canada: Cheneliere/McGraw Hill.

Hogue, W. F. (2003). *Strategic and assessment plan for distance and distributed learning at the University of South Carolina.* Retrieved October 8, 2004, from http://www.it.sc.edu/oit/docs/eLearningstrategicplan.pdf

Kearsley, G. (2000). *Online education: Learning and teaching in cyberspace.* Belmont, CA: Wadsworth/Thomson Learning.

Kennedy, D. M. (2002). Dimensions of distance: A comparison of classroom education and distance education. *Nurse Education Today, 22,* 409–416.

Kiernan, V. (2003). A survey documents growth in distance education in late 1990s. *The Chronicle of Higher Education, 49*(48). Retrieved October 6, 2004, from http://chronicle.com/prm/weekly/v49/i48/48a02802.htm

Moore, M. G. (1989). Three types of interaction. *American Journal of Distance of Education, 3*(2), available at http://www.ajde.com, retrieved March 28, 2002.

Moore, M. G., & Kearsley, G. (1996). *Distance education: A systems view.* Belmont, CA: Wadsworth.

O'Neil, C. A., Fisher, C. A., & Newbold, S. K. (Eds.). (2004). Course management methods. In *Developing an online course: Best practices for nurse educators* (pp. 97–124). New York: Springer.

Palloff, R., & Pratt, K. (1999). *Building learning communities in cyberspace: Effective strategies for the online classroom.* San Francisco: Jossey-Bass.

PART 3

Where Are We Going With Distance Education?

CHAPTER 13

Program Innovations and Technology in Nursing Education: Are We Moving Too Quickly?

Marilyn H. Oermann

Over the last few years, nursing education has received much attention by the media and public. First there was the nursing shortage and how schools of nursing were responding, and then came the faculty shortage and what nursing programs were doing about a shortage of educators. Nursing education is no longer invisible—these shortages have impressed on the public the importance of nurses and the programs that prepare them. What better publicity could we have asked for? Nursing education has always been a leader among the health professions in developing innovative programs, using technology for teaching and for delivering education to those who otherwise would not have access, and responding quickly to changing societal health needs. Until recently, though, most of our educational innovations were known only within nursing. Not any more. The attention given by the media to the nursing and faculty shortages has highlighted our innovations to prepare more nurses and deliver education to students across geographical boundaries while considering their work and family responsibilities.

Many nursing faculty have embraced technology, rushed to develop online courses and programs, and marketed their courses and programs similar to selling other products. Some of the current efforts are direct responses by schools to the nursing shortage. But are we clear about the future directions of our programs? Do we know where we are going with these efforts? The purpose of this chapter is to examine selected trends in distance education in nursing and future directions. Schools of nursing need to be clear about the goals and intended outcomes of their programs and whether a particular innovation or technology should be used considering those outcomes and their resources. Faculty are responsible for maintaining the quality of their programs and assuring the public of that quality. Our innovations in delivering programs and teaching students cannot sacrifice the quality of the education. Although this has always been important, it is more so now because nursing is the focus of media coverage and of interest to the public.

INNOVATIONS IN NURSING PROGRAMS: ONE RESPONSE TO THE NURSING SHORTAGE

According to the projections from the U.S. Bureau of Labor Statistics (2004), more than 1 million additional registered nurses (RNs) will be needed by 2012. In those reports, nursing is identified as the occupation with the largest job growth. Low student enrollment in earlier years, an aging nursing workforce, more elderly persons requiring health care, and more complex needs of patients in hospitals and other care settings have contributed to the demands for more RNs. For many years nursing programs had to market their programs vigorously to maintain enrollment, and those years have clearly had an impact on the current shortage. With the growing interest in nursing as a career and the demand for nurses, enrollments in entry-level nursing programs have increased significantly (American Association of Colleges of Nursing [AACN], 2003b; National League for Nursing, 2003). However, these increases will not compensate for the low enrollment over the last decade or for the number of nurses who are retiring.

Schools of nursing have responded to the nursing shortage by developing new and innovative programs and using technology to deliver those programs to students, many of whom otherwise would not have access to nursing education. Although there are many initiatives ongoing at individual schools of nursing, the use of distance education by more and more schools to deliver their programs to students is particularly notable.

Distance Education

Distance education in nursing continues to develop at a phenomenal pace. It is becoming difficult to find a nursing program, public or private, that does not offer courses for distance education or at least some form of online instruction. Though some faculty are concerned that distance education has initiated the demise of the traditional classroom and nursing program, others view it as creating an opportunity for nursing to prepare students across geographic boundaries, relieving shortages in rural and other areas where there are no schools of nursing. Distance education and Web-based technologies allow for career advancement for nurses no matter where they live and offer nursing education that is flexible and takes into consideration work and family responsibilities. Many students cannot attend a traditional nursing program but can learn at a time and place convenient for them.

The flexibility inherent in distance education programs makes them attractive to RNs who want to advance their education yet are unable to do so for the same reasons as students who cannot pursue an entry-level program. Many distance programs in nursing are intended for RN-BSN students (Grumet & Gilbert, 2004). Although these programs do not ease the shortage in terms of numbers of graduates, they raise the educational level of nurses, which meets yet another need—preparing more nurses at the baccalaureate and higher levels. Distance education programs for RNs in the future may shift more toward RN-MSN tracks, preparing nurses for advanced nursing practice rather than offering them bachelor's degrees in nursing. Along the same line, distance education provides a means of offering accelerated BSN-PhD programs to nurses in areas where there are no doctoral nursing programs and for specialized areas of nursing education that are not available in a particular school.

Faculty Decisions About Distance Education

Many schools of nursing now offer distance education courses, and some have complete programs online. However, with greater choices for students, schools may focus their distance education on areas of nursing in which they have particular and known expertise. Or they may offer for distance education only those courses or programs in which enrollment is typically too small for an on-campus program such as a post-master's certificate in transcultural nursing or courses in end-of-life care.

Faculty need to decide which courses, clinical majors, and programs are best offered through distance education and online learning and which should remain face-to-face. Many of the outcomes of courses taught in a traditional classroom environment can be replicated in an online course, but the faculty time to develop and implement an online course, give prompt feedback to learners, maintain communication with students, and work with clinical preceptors may exceed the time available, particularly considering faculty's scholarship and clinical practice commitments. Some schools may decide not to offer any distance education courses and instead remain an on-campus-only school of nursing. Others may use distance education only for highly specialized areas of content. It is unlikely that schools of nursing will have sufficient faculty and resources in the future to continue to offer a full range of courses, majors, and programs that often overlap with other schools.

Student Recruitment

Distance education creates a new type of competition for schools of nursing. In early years, many programs competed for students mainly in the local and regional areas. However, now with online courses and programs, the competition for students extends beyond any geographic boundaries, and some schools have invested much effort and resources in recruiting nursing students to their online programs. In a highly competitive e-learning market, institutions need to specialize in meeting particular niches in that market (Gallagher, 2003). Nursing programs that focus their distance education on specialized areas of nursing may find it easier to recruit students in future years. Even with programs that meet a niche in nursing education, though, schools will need to invest resources on marketing and ensuring high quality of their courses.

Student Decision Making—Can They Assess Quality?

With distance education students can search nationwide for courses, programs, and faculty that meet their particular educational needs. Many prospective nursing students already shop around for the best program for them, and this will likely increase as more distance programs become available. However, prospective students may be unaware of differences in quality across these programs and standards for evaluating their quality. In nursing education we have developed already a buyer-beware situation, with students completing distance programs of questionable quality and outcomes. Schools of nursing need to take an active role in educating prospective students about how to judge the quality of an online nursing program, which is different from selecting a Web-based course for personal development.

Outcomes of Courses and Programs

With the proliferation of online nursing courses and programs and other distance education methods, research is needed to establish the outcomes of those courses and programs in areas other than knowledge and student and teacher satisfaction. Chaffin and Maddux (2004) suggested from their review of the literature that online courses are effective for teaching theory, critical thinking, and clinical skills and for fostering international collaboration. Much of the research though has been done in one setting only and with small groups of students; more controlled studies across settings are needed to guide our decision making about courses, their design, and student activities in them.

Maintaining Quality

The other pressing need in nursing education is to examine and maintain the quality of online courses and other forms of distance education. There are faculty who place their PowerPoint presentations on Blackboard, WebCT, and other course management systems; they then add a few notes to accompany those visuals and label it an online course. Most nursing faculty do not have the educational background or skills to develop an online course. Instructional designers are needed on-site in schools of nursing or as consultants to work with nursing faculty to develop online courses and activities and other methods for distance education. Schools of nursing also need systematic assessment processes in place to ensure the quality of their online courses and that they are as rigorous as the ones offered in a traditional format.

PROGRAM INNOVATIONS ... BUT NO ONE TO TEACH

As schools of nursing move forward with program innovations and new initiatives, they face limited numbers of faculty to teach in those programs, a situation likely to worsen. More students are applying to nursing programs than in previous years, but there are not enough faculty to teach those students and in some programs not enough clinical settings, classrooms, and learning laboratories to increase enrollment. Last year nearly 16,000 qualified applicants to baccalaureate nursing programs alone were unable to be admitted because there were not enough faculty or instructional resources (AACN, 2003b).

One main reason for the current faculty shortage is that more educators are retiring than are being replaced in schools of nursing. The mean age for master's-prepared faculty is 48.8 years and for nurse educators with doctoral degrees 53.3 years (AACN, 2003a). Schools of nursing have had increases in their graduate program enrollments, but many students complete those programs part-time and assume roles in clinical and other settings for higher salaries. This has resulted in a pool that is too small to replace faculty who are retiring.

Strategies to Address Faculty Shortage

The faculty shortage is likely to continue for years to come, and schools need to develop other strategies for educating nursing students. Through partnerships with clinical agencies, advanced practice nurses can teach students at different program levels and can coordinate preceptor experiences in that setting, with the school supplementing their salaries or providing adjunct appointments, reduced tuition, continuing education, and cooperative programs for staff, among others. Partnerships provide a way of pooling resources and talents and sharing responsibility for preparing future nurses (Barger & Das, 2004). Partnerships with clinical agencies only work though if the school adequately prepares those advanced practice nurses, preceptors, and other clinicians for teaching roles and develops clear systems for communicating with them.

Some schools are asking retired faculty to teach part-time, conduct program evaluation, advise students, and carry out other roles, relieving faculty of those responsibilities so they can focus on new program initiatives. Teaching in schools of nursing needs to be attractive to potential faculty who may not want to pursue research and scholarship but are expert clinicians. Strong clinical tracks with contracts, promotions, and merit raises comparable to tenure line make the role more attractive and create a stable faculty group.

Release time for faculty to gain expertise in developing courses for distance education, learning new instructional technologies, and redesigning courses and experiences for an online environment is a way of developing innovations without burdening existing faculty. Release time might range from a semester without a teaching assignment to one without committee work depending on the needs of the school and faculty.

Distance education provides a mechanism for addressing the faculty shortage across a geographic area if schools are willing to share courses, instructional resources, and faculty. Schools with insufficient numbers of faculty can develop collaborative arrangements in which they share distance education courses or faculty, or new programs can be established for this purpose. Baumlein (2004) suggested that nursing programs that have similar curricula should develop online consortia rather than each school offering the same courses. Issues with tuition costs, residency requirements, and other university requirements need to be resolved before these collaborative arrangements can be implemented.

New Faculty Roles

As increasing numbers of faculty teach at a distance, new faculty roles are developing. Nurse educators are now able to teach in "virtual schools of nursing" or online courses for multiple nursing programs either in addition to their current positions or as a full-time commitment. Faculty conflicts of interest may arise in some of these situations with schools competing for the same distance education students. How do faculty with multiple teaching alliances decide where to place most of their emphasis in teaching? Conflicts can result in how faculty allocate their limited time and resources when teaching in multiple programs.

Nurse educators might choose to become "virtual adjunct" faculty, teaching for multiple distance education programs, but will the quality of nursing education be threatened by the presence of too large a number of part-time faculty? Increases in adjunct faculty positions, even if online, also limit the prospects of faculty members who want full-time and more permanent teaching positions (Carnevale, 2004).

Preparation for Educator Role

The faculty shortage is not only in terms of sheer numbers of educators to teach nursing students. The shortage also includes faculty with knowledge and competencies to carry out their roles. Because of the shift of master's programs years ago to preparing advanced practice nurses instead of nurse educators, many individuals currently in teaching roles or considering faculty positions have not been prepared for the role of educator. To develop innovations and use new technologies in teaching, faculty need to know how to teach; otherwise, they cannot make careful decisions about how to use these new methods in promoting learning outcomes.

More graduate programs are now offering nursing education as a track, individual courses to prepare faculty, or a post-master's certificate (Oermann, in review). This trend is important because of our need to prepare nurses for future roles as faculty and to further develop the knowledge and competencies of current educators. Courses and programs such as these can be offered through distance education to prepare faculty in regions without graduate nursing programs or where the schools of nursing lack resources to prepare for this role. Web-based courses developed in modular format can be packaged to meet individual needs of schools and health care settings for teacher development. For example, modules on clinical evaluation can be used for faculty development in a nursing program or as continuing education for individual faculty or educators in clinical settings.

Even if prepared as educators, faculty need strong mentors to foster their development as expert teachers and scholars. Many schools have strong mentoring programs for faculty research and scholarship, but mentors are equally important for developing expert teaching skills, particularly in schools that use technology to deliver their educational programs and in teaching.

TECHNOLOGY: CHANGING HOW
AND WHAT WE TEACH

Technology has changed the way we teach nursing at all levels and will continue to have an impact on how we deliver instruction and promote student learning. With technology we can build flexibility in the program, allowing students to learn when convenient for them and often in a setting of their choice, providing individualized learning opportunities, and creating simulated experiences that students would not have available in the clinical setting. Any time, any place learning will continue to be requested by students.

Technology also leads to more global schools that can provide high-quality education to an international student body. This is a developing market for nursing programs, particularly those with existing technology to deliver courses to students and nurses in other countries. Billings and colleagues (2003) described a collaborative effort between her school of nursing in the United States and the Institute of Health Sciences and Nursing in Malaysia to offer a Web-based course to prepare nurse educators for faculty and staff development positions in Malaysia. For countries without language and technology barriers, this market will be easier to develop.

Educational technology, though, requires faculty expertise not only in the technology itself but also in how to use it effectively in instruction. Most faculty will not be able to keep up with new developments in educational technology, particularly in schools with missions other than education. Administrative expectations that demand faculty expertise in using technology in their courses present challenges for faculty whose skill levels may be limited (Chaffin & Maddux, 2004). Faculty need experts in technology who serve as consultants to help them make decisions about what available technology would benefit students in a course regardless of how that course is delivered. Schools of nursing need to make careful decisions about allocating resources for technology because without use across the curriculum, the costs are not warranted.

Technology not only affects the way we teach but also influences what we teach. As new technologies are introduced into health care, students need to understand their use either for their own practice or to prepare patients for upcoming procedures and treatments. The rapid changes in technology in health care make it difficult for some nursing faculty to keep the curriculum current and prepare students for using technology in clinical practice. Partnerships with clinical agencies, task forces that include clinical experts, and similar arrangements provide a mechanism for faculty who are not involved in clinical practice to keep current with new technologies that students should learn about or develop some level of expertise in.

Simulations for Development of Technological Skills and Critical Thinking

Simulations and virtual technology are being integrated in many schools of nursing at all levels. They allow risk-free learning opportunities for students in a controlled environment (Oermann, 2004a, 2004b). With simulations and virtual technology, students can develop their psychomotor skills and practice those skills as they progress through a nursing program so that they maintain their competence. Another important use of simulations is to provide experiences for students to develop their critical thinking and problem-solving skills. Simulations also give students an opportunity to role-model interactions with patients, staff, and others in a safe environment, and arrive at decisions that are not only nursing focused. They provide an adjunct to live clinical instruction, which for many schools is important because of limited clinical experiences and settings and a shortage of faculty and preceptors to teach clinical courses (Krautscheid & Burton, 2003).

As schools allocate resources for high-fidelity human simulators and to develop patient simulation laboratories, there need to be mechanisms for integrating these within courses in the curriculum in lieu of clinical experiences. Similar to technology in general, faculty need guidance how best to use simulations in their courses. Otherwise, simulation laboratories are used by a few faculty and courses in a curriculum. In a survey of 34 nursing programs with laboratories with human patient simulators, Nehring and Lashley (2004) found they were used mainly in undergraduate physical assessment, advanced undergraduate medical-surgical, graduate physical assessment, and nurse anesthesia courses. Their survey also revealed that only 25% of the faculty in a school of nursing incorporated the available human-patient simulators in their courses. When unsure of technology, as a result, some faculty are wary and fearful of using it in their teaching (Nehring & Lashley, 2004).

One main outcome of using simulations is to foster students' clinical thinking through analysis of scenarios. Scenarios can be developed for students to apply their knowledge from one course to a simulated situation and to integrate learning from across courses as a basis for decision making. Developing and testing these scenarios take time, something that most faculty do not have.

Similar to technology use in general, before purchasing a human-patient simulator, redesigning a laboratory as a clinical learning center, or acquiring expensive technology, schools need to identify

1. how those technologies will be used in courses throughout the programs,
2. who will be responsible for preparing scenarios that guide students in developing their clinical judgment skills not just their psychomotor and technological competencies,
3. who will evaluate the effectiveness of simulated experiences on course outcomes,
4. how will faculty be prepared to use such technology in their own teaching, and
5. who will direct and maintain those laboratories.

Because of the high costs, simulation laboratories are best shared among schools of nursing and other health professions, and with clinical agencies. Collaboration across schools also helps ease the shortage of faculty to work with students in these laboratories. Peteani (2004) recommended that schools of nursing outsource simulators to cover their costs. Funding, how to maintain the technology long term, and specifics of sharing those laboratories across schools and health systems are issues that should be resolved early on.

SUMMARY

This chapter examined a few of the issues that accompany program innovations and technology in nursing education. Schools of nursing have responded to the shortage with new program development and expansion of distance education. The faculty shortage, however, both in numbers of faculty and in educators with expertise in technology and teaching in general has limited some of these efforts. Technology has affected how we teach and what we teach in nursing, and schools are faced with how to keep faculty current with changing technology in education and health care. As schools move forward with program innovations, distance education, and simulated laboratories, among other new developments, there are issues that should be addressed early in the decision making. The time is here for schools to decide on the programs they will offer, how they will deliver them to students, and what types of teaching methods and technologies students will find in their school of nursing.

REFERENCES

American Association of Colleges of Nursing (AACN). (2003a, May). *AACN white paper: Faculty shortages in baccalaureate and graduate nursing programs: Scope of the problem and strategies for expanding the supply.* Retrieved February 6, 2004, from http://www.aacn.nche.edu/Publications/WhitePapers/FacultyShortages.htm

American Association of Colleges of Nursing. (2003b). *Thousands of students turned away from the nation's nursing schools despite sharp increase in enrollment.* Retrieved November 6, 2004, from http://www.aacn.nche.edu/Media/NewsReleases/enrl03.htm

Barger, S. E., & Das, E. (2004). An academic-service partnership: Ideas that work. *Journal of Professional Nursing, 20*(2), 97–102.

Baumlein, G. (2004). Internet-based education. In L. Caputi & L. Engelmann (Eds.), *Teaching nursing: The art and science* (Vol. 1, pp. 248–270). Glen Ellyn, IL: College of DuPage Press.

Berlin, L., Stennett, J., & Bednash, G. (2003). *Enrollment and graduations in baccalaureate and graduate programs in nursing.* Washington, DC: American Association of Colleges of Nursing.

Billings, D., Kolandai, L., Li, I. C. M., Devi, S., Rudie, G., Mazani, M., & Paramasuvarum, S. (2003). International distance learning collaboration to prepare nurse educators in Malaysia. In M. H. Oermann & K. Heinrich (Eds.), *Annual Review of Nursing Education* (Vol. 1, pp. 267–279). New York: Springer.

Carnevale, D. (2004, April 30). For online adjuncts, a seller's market. *Chronicle of Higher Education, 50*(34), A31.

Chaffin, A. J., & Maddux, C. D. (2004). Internet teaching methods for use in baccalaureate nursing education. *CIN: Computers Informatics Nursing, 22,* 132–142.

Gallagher, R. (2003). *The next 20 years: How is online distance learning likely to evolve?* 2003 University Council for Educational Administration 88th Annual Conference, March 28–30, 2003. Chicago, Illinois.

Grumet, B. R., & Gilbert, C. (2004). An overview of trends in nursing education. In M. H. Oermann & K. Heinrich (Eds.), *Annual review of nursing education* (Vol. 2, pp. 3–18). New York: Springer.

Krautscheid, L., & Burton, D. (2003, December). *Technology in nursing education. Oregon education-based technology needs assessment: Expanding nursing education capacity.* Retrieved November 5, 2004, from http://www.oregon centerfornursing.org/about/Tech_Assessment.pdf

National League for Nursing. (2003). *NLN 2002–2003 Survey of RN Nursing Programs indicates positive upward trends in the nursing workforce supply.* New York: Author.

Nehring, W. M., & Lashley, F. R. (2004). Current use and opinions regarding human patient simulators in nursing education: An international survey. *Nursing Education Perspectives, 25,* 244–248.

Oermann, M. H. (2004a). Basic skills for teaching and the advanced practice nurse. In L. Joel (Ed.), *Advanced practice nursing: Essentials for role development* (pp. 398–429). Philadelphia: Davis.

Oermann, M. H. (2004b). Reflections on undergraduate nursing education: A look to the future. *Journal of Nursing Education Scholarship, 1*(1), 1–15. Available at http://www.bepress.com/ijnes/vol1/iss1/art5

Oermann, M. H. Post-master's certificate in nursing education: Strategy for preparing nursing faculty. (In review)

Peteani, L. A. (2004). Enhancing clinical practice and education with high-fidelity human patient simulators. *Nurse Educator, 29,* 25–30.

United States Bureau of Labor Statistics. (2004, February 11). Table 3c. *The 10 occupations with the largest job growth, 2002–12. Office of Occupational Statistics and Employment Projections United States Department of Labor.* Retrieved November 4, 2004, from http://www.bls.gov/news.release/ecopro. t05.htm

CHAPTER 14

Attitudes Toward Distance Education: A "Disruptive" Technology?

Robert H. Davis

Without question, nursing education has started down the distance education road. And, regardless of how you feel about it, there is no turning back. It's a one-way street that we have committed ourselves to and the only concern now is where we'll end up. In my former professional life, I was a police officer. Patrolling the rural outback of Lexington County, South Carolina, I sometimes found myself traveling a road I had not been down before. Curiosity compelled me to continue, even though I didn't know where I'd end up. On a pleasant day this was a rather fun adventure. However, on that same road in the dead of night, chasing a fleeing car at higher and higher speeds, not knowing where I was or where I was headed made me a bit uneasy. Every additional mile per hour on the speedometer, an unexpected turn, a hole in the road, or a fallen tree all could spell disaster. Even in emergent circumstances, caution was often the better part of valor. The bad guy sometimes got away, but I would live to work another day. The distance education highway is much like that road I traveled as a police officer. We have not been down this way before and there are some potential hazards ahead. We must resist the temptation to barrel recklessly and blindly ahead at top speeds, throwing caution to the wind. This chapter will consider the concept of disruptive technology and whether distance education (DE) in nursing is such a disruptive force and will then consider some of the potential implications.

DISRUPTIVE TECHNOLOGY

Clayton Christenson (2003) wrote about the concept of disruptive technologies in *The Innovator's Dilemma*. In his book, Christenson describes two different types of technology that organizations encounter and how each affects the course of the organization. In this context, technology is not limited to a machine, device, or computer program. A technology can be any force or concept that creates change in an organization. Christenson categorizes technology as either sustaining or disruptive. A sustaining technology helps an organization improve an existing product. It is usually incremental in nature but sometimes can be a radical change that has some of the characteristics of a disruptive technology. Sustaining technologies are almost always introduced by established and respected leaders in their field. Skills labs development in nursing schools is an example of a sustaining technology in nursing education. A recent example is the emergence of virtual reality and other simulation equipment in skills labs. This technology first surfaced in larger, more well-known nursing schools that showcased the improvements to attract more students and retain their places as leaders in the field of nursing education. As the equipment became more widely available and affordable, more schools began to purchase and implement the technology until the presence of simulation equipment in skills labs was no longer particularly unique. The schools that used this innovation to improve their programs and establish differentiation are now seeking other sustaining innovations to make their program unique and help them remain the perceived leaders in their field. From this example, one can see that introduction of simulation technology in nursing skills labs, although exciting and innovative, was merely a natural progression initiated by perceived industry leaders that helped sustain their place of leadership in the existing market.

Disruptive technologies are very different in nature from sustaining technologies. These innovations are initially dismissed by established industry leaders as "inferior products." Because of this initial rejection by the establishment, disruptive technologies often then find their niche in markets of little interest to the industry leaders, and gain popular acceptance, often exceeding the level of quality of the "mainstream" technology. Even though the so-called disruptive technology may never be "as good" as the established technology, at some point it begins to be viewed as "good enough," especially when factoring in the lower cost or greater convenience that are typically characteristic of a disruptive technology. Convenience often proves to be the defining characteristic and customers are willing to pay prices well above the cost of the existing technology. Christenson (2003) chronicles how the established firms then attempt to enter the market represented by the disruptive technology and, almost without exception, fail. Thus, the disruptive technology then is seen as a threat by established industries.

We might be tempted to dismiss this concept of disruptive technologies as applicable only to the business world. However, sustaining and disruptive technologies are realities in any organization, nursing and nursing education included. In fact, Christenson provides a list of established technologies and their potentially disruptive counterparts. Of interest to this discussion are two areas that made the list. Physicians are listed as an established technology with nurse practitioners being the disruptive counterpart. When evaluated by the criteria of a disruptive technology, nurse practitioners fit perfectly. The thought of nurses making medical diagnoses and having prescriptive authority was not welcomed by the medical community. But nurse practitioners soon found a niche in markets that had become largely ignored by physicians in their push toward specialization. Nurse practitioners provided quality primary care in rural and other underserved populations (Neal, 1999). Their care was more accessible and less costly than care provided by physicians. Studies began to show that care provided by NPs was "as good as" that of physicians in many cases. This has had a large disruptive effect on medicine, and nursing continues to demonstrate its competence in primary care.

"Classroom and campus-based instruction" also made Christenson's (2003) list, with its disruptive counterpart being distance education. Is distance education (DE), as Christenson alleges, really a disruptive technology? If yes, what are the implications for nursing education? These are some of the questions that will be addressed in the following pages.

First, does DE qualify as a potentially disruptive technology in nursing? There are several key characteristics or criteria necessary in evaluating an innovation as disruptive. A disruptive technology is often perceived as inferior to the existing technology (at least at first). A disruptive technology is often dismissed and shunned by industry leaders as unnecessary. Because the disruptive innovation lacks support from the usually larger industry leaders, smaller and less known competitors find a place to test and develop the new technology. This new value network is often the result of voids created by the industry leaders. The disruptive technology has attributes of value that those in the new value network desire, which creates a market for the innovation. Finally, disruptive innovations are often cheaper, simpler, smaller, and more convenient to use. Distance education in nursing will be evaluated against those criteria.

"INFERIOR" PRODUCT PERFORMANCE

Those who are reading this book are at least interested in distance education and are most likely supportive of it. However, at present, the literature suggests that DE is still viewed by both students and faculty as inferior to classroom lectures in nursing education. Complaints currently outweigh positive feedback when evaluating attitudes toward distance education in the nursing literature.

Faculty Perceptions

Negative attitudes by faculty toward DE can be categorized into two main areas along with several other less frequently cited complaints. Overwhelmingly, the chief complaint from faculty about online education concerns the increased workload associated with this form of educational delivery. Cravener (1999) appears to have completed the most comprehensive work to date in the area of nursing faculty experience with online education. Cravener found that workload issues expressed by faculty included a number of issues. In addition to general observations of increased time requirements, faculty commented on some specific areas as well. Because students can e-mail a faculty member 24 hours a day, 7 days a week, faculty find themselves faced with a much greater volume of communication from students to respond to than is possible in a traditional classroom setting. Due to lack of familiarity with the new technology, faculty find that it takes them much longer to prepare for the same presentation in an online format than it would in a traditional classroom or lecture format. Faculty also cite that they had to spend additional time orienting students to the class format and the technology and procedures that would be used. Ryan, Carlton, and Ali (1999) noted faculty concern with workload in teaching online courses, especially those involving asynchronous activities (communication not conducted in real time). In a previous article, Cravener (1998) noted that faculty are hesitant to participate in teaching online courses because they do not get the support and credit they feel they deserve for the additional work needed to teach the course. Although it is outside the scope of this chapter, it must be mentioned that numerous authors addressed the issue of support, recognition, and reward for faculty teaching online course work (Billings,

1999, 2000; Lewis, Watson, & Newfield, 1997; Milstead & Nelson, 1998). This is an area for further study and conversation, as it will greatly influence faculty attitudes toward participation in online education.

In addition to the workload issue, Cravener (1999) also identified some negative responses from faculty related to issues of communication. Faculty said that online modalities created a lack of visual and nonverbal cues that complicated and detracted from their communication. They also felt that online communication methods were more formal and less spontaneous than in-person communication. Faculty felt that online courses inhibited their ability to improvise as they were accustomed to doing in the classroom. Finally in the area of communication, Cravener's (1998) earlier work identified that faculty's feelings of self-worth were threatened in online courses. The basis of these feelings stemmed from the fact that faculty base a portion of their self-worth on face-to-face contact with students.

Moving on to other negative issues expressed by faculty, Cravener (1998) reported that faculty felt threatened by the newer distance education formats because it made them feel that their current methods were inadequate, insufficient, or less than optimal. They also expressed that it made them feel incompetent. Some of the other issues expressed by faculty (Cravener, 1999) were that synchronous activities could be complicated if students were in different time zones or even on different continents. Faculty were concerned that communicating across cultural boundaries could be more difficult if a student was not present in a traditional classroom. When a production team was used to develop the course for an instructor, there were fears of content and other errors as the production team generally had little knowledge of the content.

Student Perceptions

In the literature, students cite isolation, physical or technical problems, negative faculty attitudes, and communication as the biggest barriers to online education. The most frequently cited negative quality of online education reported by students is a sense or feeling of isolation. In addition to general feelings of isolation (Billings, 2000; Carlton, Ryan, & Siktberg, 1998), students expressed some more specific comments that contributed to their feelings of isolation. Ryan and colleagues (1999) included a qualitative section to their study and allowed students to express comments about their experiences. Some of the comments from students included that they felt disconnected from the class and class interaction, that there was not enough interaction and spontaneous discussion, that they missed the value of shared ideas, and that they felt "out there by myself" and increasingly anxious until they met in a real class. Next to feelings of isolation, students expressed feelings of frustration over physical or technical problems as their second most frequently cited problem with online education. Hardware and software problems were mentioned in one study (Ryan et al., 1999) and problems connecting or staying connected to the Internet was cited in several studies (Carlton et al., 1998; Ryan et al., 1999). Other comments mentioned in this area included students feeling insufficient experience with hardware and software (Carlton et al., 1998) and cost and need for technical support (Ryan et al., 1999). Another issue that surfaced in an article by Cravener (1998) was negative attitudes of faculty perceived by the students. In her article, students commented that they felt faculty did not appear to want to spend time with technology. Faculty seemed to prefer not to teach in distance formats. Students said professors made it clear they knew little about technology and that response to e-mails were slow or nonexistent. In the qualitative section of their study (Ryan et al., 1999), students expressed that they did not like everyone being able to read their comments, that they were uncertain of their progress in class, and that they felt there was no flow of communication in the class.

It is only fair to clarify that there are positive attitudes toward DE by both students and faculty. However, the solid majority of evidence in the literature currently supports a negative bias toward DE. Based on the prevalence of negative experiences with DE, it can be concluded that there is a perception that DE is currently an inferior product when compared with traditional on-campus lecture as a means of educational delivery. It would appear that DE in nursing meets the first criterion of a disruptive technology.

DISMISSAL BY MAINSTREAM LEADERS

A second characteristic of a disruptive technology is its dismissal by the established leaders of the particular industry. Christenson (2003) chronicles case after case in the development of computer disk drives. Established industry leaders passed up potential innovations, only to find that a previously insignificant competitor was able to find a use for the innovation in a more obscure market. The new company developed the drive until it became almost as good as the existing product but with greater convenience, and the existing leaders inevitably found themselves looking up at the new leaders. The literature referenced in the previous section supports this second point as well. Although some positive attitudes toward DE are reflected in the literature, most is negative. Unfortunately, very little research has been conducted looking at the attitudes of nursing school administrators and their attitudes and commitment to establishing DE as part of the curriculum. This gap in the literature may suggest an area of further research. Anecdotally, from personal conversations and informal surveys of schools at professional meetings by the author, it would appear that smaller, less known schools are more progressive in developing distance education. Larger, more established institutions appear to be much more firmly entrenched in the brick-and-mortar campus and more resistant to embracing DE. Based on the circumstantial evidence considered, DE in nursing also fulfills this second important criterion of a disruptive technology.

VALUE NETWORKS AND DESIRABLE ATTRIBUTES

The third and fourth characteristics will be considered together. Christenson (2003) describes how a disruptive technology is dismissed by the mainstream and because of that must establish itself and then grow within a newly created "value network." A value network is a context within which an organization makes all of its strategic and operational decisions, and it includes internal and external factors such as mission, goals, target market, suppliers, and so forth. Christenson chronicles how organizations often become captive to their established value network, which keeps them from responding to the threat of a disruptive technology when it arises. This occurs when an organization becomes so overly concerned about the needs of their "best" customers that they are blinded to the voids being created and also blind to competitors willing to cater to the smaller and usually less profitable markets. The preceding discussion of the literature regarding attitudes toward DE would suggest that nursing education may be captive to a value network that is not allowing it to respond to the threat of DE. Faculty, administrators, and, to a lesser extent, current students, insecure with the disruptive DE innovations, clamor for sustaining innovation that will keep the on-campus setting intact. Not able to establish itself initially within traditional mainstream nursing education, DE developed a new value network in which to grow and develop. Traditional nursing education values customers (aka students) who are willing to come to a classroom on a weekly basis, during daytime hours, for the duration of a quarter or semester. Some sustaining technologies that have been in the evolution of education have expanded the customer base with, for example, night and weekend classes and the intensive course (courses that meet for consecutive days). But DE seems to have initially created its value network in a market not particularly of interest to traditional education. Where DE established itself was in the world of continuing education and among degree-seeking candidates who did not have convenient access to a traditional campus. Long before many nurses ever used any type of distance education in a college setting, they had grown accustomed to using computer based education (CBE) learning in the hospital for in-service training. Although not "distance" in the way we think of it today, the training modules had the hallmarks of today's DE: available almost any time of day or night at the learner's convenience, and self-paced. It wasn't long before this training became available at terminals in the nursing units, and continuing education units (CE) began to be offered using these formats as well. CE is the other part of this new value market. Both in-service training and CE appealed to the same target audience: working nurses, established in their careers, with other life responsibilities, who needed convenient, flexible, and affordable educational opportunities. Those demographics were not part of mainstream nursing education's value network. The early CBE courses at hospitals and CEU courses were, by most standards, inferior to lectures given by experts. However, the point is that DE had created a value network in which to develop and grow, a value network that was also free from the interest of traditional education. In this fertile value network, technology improved, and nurses began to become accustomed to education delivered this way. Although arguably inferior to traditional methods of education and largely dismissed by mainstream nursing education, DE had found a new value network in which to grow and improve, offering education that was convenient and flexible, two values of tremendous importance to working nurses. Once again, DE meets several more criteria required to be considered a disruptive technology.

COST AND CONVENIENCE

Finally, a disruptive technology is usually cheaper, simpler, smaller, or more convenient to use (by the customer)—or all of the above—than is the existing technology. On most accounts, DE is not cheaper than traditional education. A credit hour is a credit hour and generally costs the same regardless of how it is delivered. In fact, some academic institutions charge more for a DE course because it is more time-intensive to prepare and deliver. As far as being easier to use, some would argue with that as well. Where DE does fulfill this last criterion is that it is more convenient than traditional methods of educational delivery. In the case of Internet-mediated delivery, course notes and lectures can often be accessed anytime and anywhere and completed at a pace more individualized to the learner

(Kenny, 2002; Wambach et al., 1999). In many of the organizations and industries described by Christenson (2003), customers within the new value networks were often willing to pay more for the disruptive technology if the convenience was substantially better than the current technology. Thus, DE does fulfill this final criterion for establishing it as a disruptive innovation in nursing education.

If DE truly is a disruptive force in nursing education, there are some major implications that must be recognized and addressed. Throughout his book, Christenson (2003) frequently refers to disruptive innovations as threats. Christenson documented the outcomes of organizations that were faced with disruptive technologies. The results are very consistent when applied to organizations of varying size and type. If the model holds true to DE in nursing education, many programs potentially face some difficult times ahead. In every case documented by Christenson, organizations that did not recognize the disruptive threat early and adapt quickly and appropriately lost their place as leaders in their respective industry and many did not survive at all. Does this mean that nursing schools will be closing their doors in large numbers? Most likely not. However, it may mean that schools clinging tightly to the traditional delivery of on-campus lectures may see declining enrollment despite the nursing shortage and increased interest in nursing. It may also mean that established schools long respected as the "premier" academic institutions in nursing may be replaced by schools that are not considered among the "elite." As an administrator reading this article, consider how your organization will respond to this disruptive threat. This may present an opportunity for you to emerge as a prominent force in what most likely will be a new field of leaders in nursing education. Faculty should begin discussions at their schools to raise the awareness of the coming changes and begin building skills in DE and seeking out experiences that allow their organizations to develop skills in this method of delivery.

CONCLUSION

As nursing educators, we are on the road toward distance education's becoming the norm. So far, the ride has been relatively uneventful, but if DE is in fact a disruptive technology, the road may get a little rough for some. There is even the potential for some serious accidents. DE fits most of the criteria of a disruptive force. Initially dismissed and frowned upon by most nursing educators, it established itself in a new value network of nurses using it for in-service education and CEUs. Initially inferior as an educational delivery method, it developed in its new value network, and has almost reached the status of "good enough" when compared to traditional classroom teaching. Considered good enough by many, customers are willing to pay for the new product because of the convenience and flexibility it offers. As is typical of disruptive technologies in other industries, DE in nursing has the potential to change the face of nursing education dramatically. It's a road we have started down and we cannot turn around.

As more of our customers (students) come to expect and demand education delivered in distance formats, those institutions that recognize this fact now and work hard to develop quality distance education can expect to benefit significantly, as students increasingly will choose those programs over traditional classroom-based programs. These same institutions most likely will find they are becoming the new leaders in nursing education, replacing those that choose to deny or ignore this disruptive force. One hopes this discussion will allow nursing schools and colleges to see DE in a different light. DE is not just a novel educational adjunct. It is a powerful and potentially disruptive force that nursing education must face and decide what to do with. To ignore or deny the challenge is to risk the fate of many other organizations that have chosen similarly. Their names are not remembered because they ceased to exist. The hope is that this chapter will prompt many educators and administrators to evaluate the place of DE in their programs and use it to prosper and to educate many more generations of aspiring nurses.

REFERENCES

Billings, D. M. (1999). The next generation distance education: Beyond access and convenience. *Journal of Nursing Education, 38,* 246–247.

Billings, D. M. (2000). A framework for assessing outcomes and practices in Web-based courses in nursing. *Journal of Nursing Education, 39*(2), 60–67.

Carlton, K. H., Ryan, M. E., & Siktberg, L. L. (1998). Designing courses for the Internet: A conceptual approach. *Nurse Educator, 23*(3), 45–50.

Christenson, C. M. (2003). *The innovator's dilemma.* New York: HarperBusiness.

Cravener, P. (1998). A psychosocial systems approach to faculty development programs. *The Technology Source.* Retrieved December 5, 2002, from http://ts.mivu.org/default.asp?show=article&id=68

Cravener, P. A. (1999). Faculty experiences with providing online courses: Thorns among roses. *Computers in Nursing, 17*(1), 42–47.

Kenny, A. (2002). Online learning: Enhancing nurse education? *Journal of Advanced Nursing, 38,* 127–135.

Leasure, A. R., Davis, L., & Thievon, S. L. (2000). Comparison of student outcomes and preferences in a traditional vs. World Wide Web-based baccalaureate nursing research course. *Journal of Nursing Education, 39,* 149–154.

Lewis, D., Watson, J. E., & Newfield, S. (1997). Implementing instructional technology: Strategies for success. *Computers in Nursing, 15,* 187–190.

Milstead, J. A., & Nelson, R. (1998). Preparation for an online asynchronous university doctoral course: Lessons learned. *Computers in Nursing, 16,* 247–258.

Neale, J. (1999). Nurse practitioners and physicians: A collaborative practice. *Clinical Nurse Specialist, 13,* 252–258.

Ryan, M., Carlton, K. H., & Ali, N. S. (1999). Evaluation of traditional classroom teaching methods versus course delivery via the World Wide Web. *Journal of Nursing Education, 38,* 272–277.

Wambach, K., Boyle, D., Hagemaster, J., Teel, C., Langner, B., Fazzone, P., et al. (1999). Beyond correspondence, video conferencing, and voice mail: Internet-based master's degree courses in nursing. *Journal of Nursing Education, 38,* 267–271.

Appendix: Sources for Online Education

American Nurses Association Continuing Education:
http://nursingworld.org/ce/cehome.cfm

This organization offers free continuing education for its members, ranging from 1.2 to 3.3 contact hours on topics such as the Code of Ethics, needlestick safety, immunizations, and home health care classification systems. There is a CE tracker that identifies the large extent of available continuing-education options via a search tool. This resource of selected online continuing-education independent study modules (ISMs) is offered to nurses who are interested in broadening their knowledge of the changing field of health care. In addition, an archive of expired ISMs is available for free at http://nursingworld.org/mods/archive/home.cfm, but without contact hour availability. A biweekly poll on the ANA Web site recorded that members earn contact hours for continuing education through print publications (35.97%), online (54.93%), and at conferences (71.64%). (Accessed 2/25/05.)

CE Connection:
http://www.nursingcenter.com/prodev/ce_online.asp

This site lists courses by nursing specialty, clinical topic, journal names, and type of media (offering articles and multimedia options); and in a variety of settings. There appear to be hundreds of offerings and the pricing ranges from $13.95 for one contact hour to $16.95 for 2 contact hours. However, you can buy a yearly subscription (CE Saver) for $29.95

and take up to 100 contact hours. The content is relevant for a wide group of nursing practitioners of all levels and backgrounds.

Homestead Schools:
http://www.homesteadschools.com/Nursing/

Credentialing through the American Nurses Credentialing Center's Commission on Accreditation (ANCC); price range: $20 for 2 contact hours to $65.95 for 30 contact hours. Online requirements: Microsoft Internet Explorer version 5.0 or higher; Netscape version 4.6 or higher; AOL versions 4.0 or 5.0. Wide range of topics offered: clinically focused (e.g., women's health, viral hepatitis, wound care) to management (e.g., stress management, nursing tips, Spanish, substance abuse).

Medscape: http://www.medscape.com/homepage

Medscape offers free, continuously updated continuing-education activities for physicians and other health professionals that are approved by the Accreditation Council for Continuing Medical Education (ACCME), and developed by ACCME-accredited organizations. Articles are available to read, test answers are posted, evaluation completed, and CME credit hours and accompanying certificate are posted.

Nursing Spectrum: http://www.nursingspectrum.com/
ContinuingEducation/NSSelfStudy/index.cfm

This site offers some free monthly continuing education if processed online as well as a broad spectrum of other continuing-education courses at a price ranging from $8 and up. Unlimited access to the courses is available for a one-time yearly price of $29.99. Accreditation is through ANCC and AACN. There is a wide variety of self-study modules to choose from in many clinical specialty and topic areas.

Sigma Theta Tau International:
http://www.nursingsociety.org/education/ceonline.html

Sigma Theta Tau International's online distance-education activities are designed to advance clinical reasoning, decision making, and judgment of practicing nurses. Case studies and articles are $10/course for members and $12/course for nonmembers. Modules are available at individually determined costs. Continuing-education activities at this site are accredited by the ANCC.

Thomson American Health Consultants (AHC): http://www.ce-web.com/gindex.php

Accredited as a provider of continuing education in nursing by the ANCC, offers many programs targeted more at primary care practitioners, approximate cost is $10/contact hour. Course vary by specialty area (17 specialties identified), and 35 topic areas that have courses ranging from 1 to 18 per topic area.

Wild Iris Medical Education: http://www.nursingceu.com

Read a course, take a test, and print out the certificate. Accredited by ANCC and American Association of Critical Care Nurses (AACCN), these courses are claimed to be valid in all 50 states. The cost is approximately $10/contact hour. Six courses listed for nursing in infection control, child abuse, standards of safe nursing practices, and HIV/AIDS prevention. The free directory of online continuing education nurse CEU. com offers free CEU courses at http://www.nurseceu.com/free.htm.

For most of these sites for online continuing education the majority of offerings are self-study modules and participants are required to pass a test (70%–80% passing rates) and complete an evaluation form to receive certification of contact hours. There is an abundance of options to choose from for nurses desiring to pursue continuing education online.

Index